AIDS

BETWEEN
SCIENCE
AND POLITICS

—

PETER PIOT

AIDS
BETWEEN
SCIENCE
AND POLITICS

TRANSLATED BY LAURENCE GAREY

COLUMBIA UNIVERSITY PRESS
NEW YORK

Columbia University Press
Publishers Since 1893
New York   Chichester, West Sussex
cup.columbia.edu
Adapted from *Le sida dans le monde: Entre science et politique*
Copyright © 2011 ODILE JACOB, Paris
Translation © 2015 Columbia University Press
All rights reserved

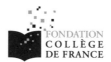

Columbia University Press wishes to express its appreciation for assistance
given by the Fondation du Collège de France and the Agence Française
de Développement toward the cost of publishing this book.

Library of Congress Cataloging-in-Publication Data
Piot, Peter, 1949- author.
[Sida dans le monde. English]
AIDS between science and politics / Peter Piot ; translated by Laurence Garey.
p. ; cm.
Includes bibliographical references and index.
Revised and updated translation of: Le sida dans le monde: entre science et
politique / Peter Piot.
Paris : Odile Jacob, c2011.
ISBN 978-0-231-16626-3 (cloth : alk. paper) — ISBN 978-0-231-53877-0 (ebook)
I. Title.
[DNLM: 1. Acquired Immunodeficiency Syndrome. 2. Government Programs.
3. Human Rights. 4. Politics. 5. Socioeconomic Factors. 6. World Health. WC 503]
RA643.8
362.19697'92—dc23
2014026530

Columbia University Press books are printed on permanent
and durable acid-free paper.
This book is printed on paper with recycled content.
Printed in the United States of America

c 10 9 8 7 6 5 4 3 2 1

Jacket design by Chris Sergio

References to websites (URLs) were accurate at the time of writing.
Neither the author nor Columbia University Press is responsible for URLs
that may have expired or changed since the manuscript was prepared.

In memory of Joep Lange and Jacqueline van Tongeren

CONTENTS

TRANSLATOR'S NOTE

AIDS is a hot topic. It is a global phenomenon, like nothing that came before it, and recognizes neither national boundaries nor social strata. In translating a book on AIDS three years after its 2011 appearance in French I realized that I was running the risk of it being out of date by the time it was published. However, Peter Piot agreed to undertake an update as I reached the end of my translation. In this task he was assiduous, and this English version is much more than just a translation of his masterly discussion of AIDS in the world—it is a new edition with Peter's 2014 revisions.

Our work has depended on many other people too. Sarah Curran, Peter's programme manager at the London School of Hygiene and Tropical Medicine, has helped ensure that things were right up to date. At Columbia University Press Bridget Flannery-McCoy and Kathryn Schell skillfully piloted the project, which was managed by Roy Thomas.

Laurence Garey
Perroy, Switzerland
February 2014

ACKNOWLEDGMENTS

This book would never have been published without the unfailing support of Heidi, the encouragement and inspiration of Philippe Kourilsky and Pierre Corvol, and without the precious help of Laurence Garey, Sarah Curran, Helena Legido-Quigly, Gabriella Gomez, Annick Borquez, Jean-Jacques Rosat, and Marie Chéron. To work with my friend and colleague Michel Caraël is always a privilege and an intellectual adventure, and his contributions were crucial for the original French version. This book reflects the work and collective engagement of thousands of people throughout the world—too numerous to cite here. I would also like to express my gratitude toward my colleagues in UNAIDS, especially to my successor Michel Sidibé. My thoughts and gratitude go to Greet, Bram, and Sara for their caring support.

Peter Piot
London, England
February 2014

AIDS

BETWEEN
SCIENCE
AND POLITICS

—

INTRODUCTION

Misunderstanding of the present is the inevitable consequence of ignorance of the past. But a man may wear himself out just as fruitlessly in seeking to understand the past, if he is totally ignorant of the present.

—Marc Bloch[1]

This book is based on ten lectures in the "Knowledge against Poverty" series at the Collège de France in Paris from 2009 to 2010. I had the unique opportunity to reflect on my experience as scientist, clinician, founding executive director of the Joint United Nations Programme on HIV/AIDS (UNAIDS), and activist in the struggle against AIDS since the epidemic began. This experience convinced me that without a political or economic connection science brings little to people, but also that without scientific evidence and respect for human rights, politics is ineffective and can even be harmful.[2] This present book represents the English translation of that original book, but also much more. This book has been completely updated and revised to reflect the latest literature and important new topics have been added to bring the critical subject of HIV/AIDS up to date.

AIDS, the acquired immunodeficiency syndrome, was one of the disruptive events that marked the turn of the twenty-first century. The AIDS pandemic was not only disruptive for the health of millions worldwide, but also disruptive in terms of international relations, global access to new technologies, and public health policies. It profoundly altered our relationship to sexuality, doctor-patient relations, the influence of civil society in international relations, and north-south solidarity. It thrust health into the realms of national and international politics, where it rightly belongs.

Who could have predicted the worst pandemic in modern history since the Spanish influenza when, in June 1981, a syndrome of unknown origin, characterized by a rare form of pneumonia, was described in just a few lines about five white homosexual men in the United States?[3] What appeared initially as a medical curiosity was overshadowed by other events such as the election of François Mitterrand as president of France, the wedding of Prince Charles and Princess Diana, and the death of Bob Marley. I was then heavily involved in epidemiological research on sexually transmitted diseases in Africa and Belgium, but far from imagining that this new syndrome would, over more than three decades, affect some seventy million people and cause over thirty million deaths. It took a long time before the full extent of the epidemic was realized, that of an unprecedented viral infection transmitted by body fluids, including genital secretions and blood, and from mother to child. The first public reactions to AIDS were dominated by fear when faced with the litany of unavoidable death and suffering, and anxiety at the defeat of medical salvation. Until then modern medical science had seemed almighty against microbes and many even thought that infectious diseases were fully under control, at least in wealthy societies.

The first years were marked by the stigmatization of those living with the virus: homosexual men, drug users, and people with hemophilia, as well as Haitians and Africans. That era is not over: although now subtler, discrimination and stigmatization explain at least partly the gap between what is possible—greatly reduced levels of infection and deaths—and the continuing global epidemic.

The first years were marked by the stigmatization of those living with the virus: homosexual men, drug users, and people with hemophilia, as well as Haitians and Africans. That era is not over: although now subtler, discrimination and stigmatization explain at least partly the gap between what is possible—greatly reduced levels of infection and deaths—and the continuing global epidemic. Reports by UNAIDS show that considerable progress has been made after more than thirty years of the epidemic, with 12.9 million people receiving antiretroviral therapy globally at the end of 2013, resulting in a 35 percent decline in deaths between 2005 and 2012, when 1.5 million people died from AIDS. In addition, the incidence (that is, new infections of human immunodeficiency virus [HIV]) decreased by 38 percent worldwide between 2001 and 2013, with 2.1 million persons newly infected in 2013.[4]

The perception of AIDS has been that of a disease that concerns "others" and has been tainted with moral judgment and condemnation. People living with HIV have succeeded in slowly dispelling a vision dominated by evil and guilt through their activist groups, which are well connected with a coalition of young doctors and scientists, of which I was one. They are highlighting men, women, and children fighting for their right to dignity, care, and their active participation in the decision-making processes, as well as in research and in the implementation of programs.

The AIDS movement was a strong disruptive force for classic visions of public health and it deepened notions of security and human development as related to health. International solidarity came belatedly, but finally became exemplary for other global issues by the creation of novel international institutions such as UNAIDS and the Global Fund to Fight AIDS, Tuberculosis and Malaria. Support for the global AIDS response has greatly expanded to include bilateral aid, foundations, nongovernmental organizations (NGOs), and political leadership. The response to AIDS changed the world in many respects. The exceptional character of the epidemic has been recognized and the political world is engaged at the highest level. Worldwide finance for the fight against AIDS increased from a few hundred thousand dollars before 1990 to nineteen billion dollars in 2013.[5] For the first time in thirty years the epidemic has receded significantly on several continents.[6]

> The end of AIDS is not in sight, considering the large number of new infections (nearly seven thousand per day) and deaths (nearly five thousand per day). The historic successes should now encourage a redoubled effort at prevention, treatment, and research, and a long-term increase in finance.

Even so, the end of AIDS is not in sight, considering the large number of new infections (nearly seven thousand per day) and deaths (nearly five thousand per day). The historic successes should now encourage a redoubled effort at prevention, treatment, and research, and a long-term increase in finance, all the more so because we must plan for the scenario that in 2030 the fight against AIDS will cost two to three times more than it does today, at a cost of up to twenty to thirty billion dollars per year.[7] In the absence of a major technological breakthrough, such as an effective vaccine, new HIV infections could still be as many as one million in 2030. Sadly, there are black clouds on the horizon. The economic crisis and other problems, such as terrorism and climate change, also require the world's attention. Some experts estimate that we are spending too much on this epidemic at the expense of other health issues; they metamorphose AIDS into a trivial chronic disease, forgetting that thirty-four million people will sooner or later need antiretroviral treatment and that for every person under treatment in the world, nearly two new people are infected with HIV.

As is so often the case, some experts hope for simple solutions to complex problems. Whereas antiretroviral treatment reduced the transmission of HIV in serodiscordant couples by more than 95 percent, it remains to be proved that early treatment would eliminate or significantly reduce HIV transmission at the population level, given the numerous logistic and other constraints of lifelong treatment. Improving access to antiretroviral treatment remains an absolute priority to save the lives of those with HIV, and will probably contribute to reducing new infections. However, "remedicalization" of AIDS seems like a regression when faced with the difficulty of considering HIV in terms of individual and collective behavior, social and cultural change, and inequality of power and status that often determine individual behavior. The dramatic increase of HIV infections in the former Soviet Union after the fall of the Berlin wall, or in South Africa after the end of apartheid, and its continuing high incidence in many gay communities, shows that people do not weigh their odds of infection as a manager does with stock options, and that a test, a drug, or a recommendation for prevention will not suffice to stem the tide of the epidemic.

The extraordinary diversity of the epidemic requires a variety of adequate preventive measures and an ensemble of integrated programs, from male circumcision to community mobilization. They include large-scale treatment based at the local level with a clear understanding of what determines new infections, the groups most affected, and the local institutions that could be mobilized, from politicians to police. Such "combination prevention" also means decentralization and better involvement of communities in the programs, while concentrating resources on "hot spots" of the highest risk of transmission.

New strategies should also mean more influence over the structural determinants of infection. Integration or better synergy of services—such as for the treatment of sexually transmitted diseases, reproductive health, family planning, schools, and prevention of tuberculosis and HIV—could improve the efficiency of services and allow more people to have access, though we need to bear in mind that specific HIV prevention programs will remain necessary for those who are not welcome in regular health services. New interventions with antiretroviral drugs, such as pre-exposure prophylaxis with either a vaginal microbicidal gel or oral medication, are promising additions to reduce HIV transmission in highly exposed populations. The search for an HIV vaccine must continue, but will certainly demand many more years of fundamental and clinical research, just like the search for a cure, which may no longer be in the realm of science fiction.

Research is necessary and must continue to orient programs confronting the concrete practical problems of HIV transmission. Recently during a lull in a major cricket game, I was conversing with sex professionals and community workers in the shanty towns of Mumbai—a

city of some eighteen million residents—during a visit to the vast Avahan HIV prevention program. I had already visited this immense area
twenty years earlier, and I could see how the program had reduced new
HIV infections in this discriminated, high-risk population. There were
some remarkable changes among the sex workers, with new capacity
to organize themselves and access to mobile telephones and financial
transactions, with a reduction in police and customer violence, elimination of pimps, and support for their organizations. In the last decade
the global reaction to the AIDS epidemic has become an illustration
of what can be achieved when science, politics, and programs on the
ground converge. But history has also taught us the fragility of solidarity
and the possible disastrous consequences of complacency and reduced
investments. It is already more than thirty years since the first case of
AIDS was reported, and yet from a historic perspective we are only at
the beginning of the epidemic. We have no choice but to refuse the fatal-
istic view of a world with unacceptable levels of HIV infection and its
devastation, and to continue the long march toward elimination of HIV,
or at the least toward reduction to very low endemic levels until there is
an effective vaccine.[8]

> In the last decade the global reaction to the AIDS epidemic has become an
> illustration of what can be achieved when science, politics, and programs
> on the ground converge.

1

A HETEROGENEOUS AND STILL-EVOLVING EPIDEMIC

RAPID GLOBAL SPREAD

AIDS was first described in 1981, which makes it a recent historic phenomenon. Following its discovery in North America and then in Western Europe, around 1985 the epicenter was considered to be in Central Africa where the HIV infection rate was 4 or 5 percent in countries such as Zaire, Rwanda, Burundi, Uganda, and Zambia. Southern Africa, which would later experience the highest HIV infection rates in the world, was hardly affected at the time. Ten years later, in 1995, the virus had spread throughout the world with an important focus in Southeast Asia, mainly connected with commercial sex. At the beginning of the twenty-first century the epidemic spread through the former Soviet republics driven by injecting drug use. Today we are still in an unstable dynamic phase of the epidemic in certain parts of the world, such as in Eastern Europe, while it has peaked in others, such as in many African countries. In Papua New Guinea, for example, an epidemic is developing with a mainly heterosexual mode of transmission. In several sub-Saharan African countries injecting drug users and men who have sex with men are now emerging as being at high risk for HIV infection, and in Asia and Western countries there is continuing high incidence among men who have sex with men.[1]

Three elements are important when considering the evolution of an epidemic like AIDS: the number of people living with HIV (*prevalence*), the *incidence* of new infections, and the number of deaths it causes.

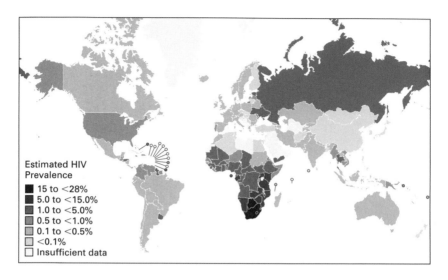

Estimated HIV
Prevalence
■ 15 to <28%
■ 5.0 to <15.0%
■ 1.0 to <5.0%
■ 0.5 to <1.0%
■ 0.1 to <0.5%
□ <0.1%
□ Insufficient data

FIGURE 1.1 WORLD MAP OF PREVALENCE OF HIV INFECTION.

DATA FROM UNAIDS (HTTP://WWW.UNAIDS.ORG), UNICEF (WWW.UNICEF.ORG),
AND THE WORLD BANK (HTTP://WWW.WORLDBANK.ORG).

Prevalence means the total number or percentage of people living with
HIV (combining old and new infections) at any given time in a population. Incidence refers to the number or rate of new infections over time,
most commonly one year. The number of people infected with HIV
reflects the sum of new infections over the years, minus the number of
deaths. In 2013 the number of people with HIV was estimated at just over
thirty-five million.[2] Overall, AIDS was the fifth leading cause of DALYs
(Disability Adjusted Life Years lost) in the world in 2010, and the first
cause of DALYs in twenty-one countries.[3] Increased access to antiretrovirals since the mid-2000s avoided millions of deaths and thus contributed
to maintaining the number of infected people at a high level. This factor
thus masked the considerable drop in new infections. New infections
in adults and children in 2013 were estimated at 2.1 million, a decline
of 38% from 2001. This drop is spectacular, even if the figure remains
high. Sub-Saharan Africa saw 1.5 million new infections in 2013, which
represents about one million fewer infections than in 2001. In South and

Southeast Asia there were approximately two hundred seventy thousand new cases in 2013, a decline of about one third since 2001. Western and Central Europe experienced an increase of HIV incidence, with twenty-nine thousand new infections, but Eastern Europe and Central Asia had the largest relative and absolute increase in HIV incidence in the world. For example, in Russia new infections rose by 50 percent between 2006 and 2011, from forty thousand to sixty thousand. In the United States new infections have remained relatively stable at around fifty thousand per year since the mid-1990s, though with a consistent increase in incidence among gay and bisexual men. The most pronounced decline in new infections since 2001 (52 percent) has occurred in the Caribbean.

More than any other figure, deaths illustrate the drama of AIDS: 1.5 million people died in 2013 in spite of the existence of antiretrovirals. The majority of these deaths occurred in sub-Saharan Africa, where AIDS is the first cause of death in about half the countries. In Europe and the United States twenty-seven thousand people died from AIDS in 2013, most of whom could have been saved if they had had access to early diagnosis and appropriate treatment.

HOW ARE HIV NUMBERS ESTIMATED?

How can we estimate the number of people infected with HIV, since tests are not implemented systematically on all populations? To estimate the extent of a disease, infection and risk are constant challenges in public health. There is a complex worldwide epidemiological survey that probably provides better public health data for AIDS than for most other conditions. Indeed, since the end of the 1980s systematic surveys of the prevalence of HIV antibody in pregnant women presenting at prenatal clinics are held, using a standardized methodology developed by the Joint United Nations Programme on HIV/AIDS (UNAIDS) and the World Health Organization (WHO). They are confidential, anonymous, and repeated every two years in the same clinics, but not with the same patients. The results allow an estimation of the infection rate in the sexually active heterosexual population. The aim is to establish trends (increase, decrease, or stability), rather than an absolute number, to facilitate organization of prevention, and anticipate needs for treatment or support for affected people.

Besides a number of logistical challenges and inadequate resources for epidemiological surveillance, estimating the level and spread of HIV infection in a large population is complicated by at least two factors. The first is the reality that HIV is not evenly distributed in a population, with some individuals and subgroups being at greater risk than others, making nationwide estimates more hazardous, as neither the burden of infection, nor the size of the groups at higher risk, are known in many countries (compounded by the fact that in some countries it is very difficult to work with certain populations as they are illegal, such as homosexual men). Specific surveys are necessary to estimate HIV prevalence in such populations. A second more recent challenge for estimating new infections is that more infected people are surviving due to antiretrovirals. The success of a program for treating AIDS is measured by a fall in mortality and therefore also by an increase in people living with HIV. Conversely, falling numbers of infected people may indicate an increase in deaths, or a long-term decrease in new infections. So, paradoxically, for at least one generation we can only hope for a decrease in new infections but an increased number of people living with HIV.

Beyond the absolute number and distribution of infections in given regions over time, national AIDS programs seek to understand which groups are affected by recent infection, as this is where efforts for HIV prevention should be focused. However, sentinel surveillance of HIV detects people whose infection may date from years earlier, which is not ideal for early prevention of infection, though it remains useful to estimate needs for antiretroviral treatment. The major problem is the absence of a reliable biological test to measure the incidence of recent HIV infections in large-scale surveys. Such a test would be particularly important to estimate whether prevention has an impact or not, or if it is targeting the groups most at risk.

HIV infection rates among young people may be a proxy for incidence in their age group, as infections through sex or injecting drug use are likely to be recent. Nevertheless extrapolating HIV prevalence in young pregnant women to the general population must be adjusted with care as we might overestimate the prevalence among other women of the same age in the general population, as well as among men, since particularly in Africa women are infected at a much younger age than men.

In spite of data from sentinel surveillance and behavioral and serological surveys it remains difficult to estimate national HIV prevalence even in countries with well-functioning systems. When new data and better methods become available estimates are updated, sometimes generating controversy or even conspiracy theories. For example, in 2008 the Centers for Disease Control (CDC) in the United States, which have access to thousands of data banks, had to adjust the HIV prevalence estimates for 2006 and recognize that 1.1 million people were HIV-positive, higher than had previously been estimated.[4] And in 2007 UNAIDS announced a major reduction in its estimates of the number of people living with HIV in India from five to 2.7 million when new data became available from a much larger number of epidemiological surveillance sites than before.

Reliance on complex statistical models is indispensable for obtaining the best estimates and predicting future evolution. UNAIDS and WHO rely heavily on a reference group of independent experts, of whom most are not directly involved in surveys. This group developed the methodology for the estimates and the relevant software. In most countries there are committees of national and international experts who examine local data. National estimates are made about every two years and the data are integrated with a worldwide bank run by UNAIDS and WHO. An alternative methodology, the Global Burden of Disease Study 2010 by the Institute for Health Metrics and Evaluation (Cause of Death Ensemble

---

In spite of data from sentinel surveillance and behavioral and serological surveys it remains difficult to estimate national HIV prevalence even in countries with well-functioning systems. When new data and better methods become available estimates are updated, sometimes generating controversy or even conspiracy theories.

model), which incorporates mortality for all causes, generated mortality estimates close to those published by UNAIDS.[5] HIV estimates can be politically highly sensitive, and countries such as Russia, China, India, and South Africa at some point challenged the UNAIDS figures, though without providing alternative evidence.

The future of the HIV epidemic depends on numerous unknowns and no model can fully determine the extent of long-term changes, either in prevention or treatment. Thus, in 1990 the worst case scenario the WHO envisaged for 2000, using the EPI Model computer program, was that fifteen to twenty-five million people would be infected with HIV throughout the world, which unfortunately proved to be millions short.[6]

GENERALIZED AND CONCENTRATED EPIDEMICS

Generalized epidemics are de facto those resulting from heterosexual transmission in the general population, as in sub-Saharan Africa, Haiti, Cambodia, or Papua New Guinea. Most countries experience *concentrated* epidemics, where HIV is associated with certain high-risk groups. In the Americas, Europe, and Australia these are mainly gay men, but in Eastern Europe around 50 percent are drug users. Paradoxically we sometimes have better figures for sub-Saharan Africa than Europe or other continents because it is easier to measure a phenomenon when it is common than when it is rare or very rare, such as in China.

In more than thirty countries, especially in Africa, random sample surveys of HIV infection in the general population have been performed, often in conjunction with existing demographic and health surveys. This approach should provide more representative estimates, but is onerous, costing seven to fifteen million dollars for a population of fifteen to twenty million, and cannot be repeated often. However, population surveys on HIV prevalence are also not without problems. For example, the rate of nonparticipation by men in such national surveys varies from 5 to 15 percent, making results difficult to interpret, the more so because groups most exposed to HIV, such as truck drivers, migrant works, soldiers, or sex workers, are systematically underrepresented, resulting in an underestimation of infection rates. Thus, in general, national population surveys gave infection rates slightly lower than those in pregnant women.[7] For example, in Lesotho estimates from pregnant women were 26.5 percent but 24 percent in a national household survey. In South Africa the differences were particularly great (29 versus 17 percent). Which figure is closer to reality? Surveys based on samples from the general population often do not include people who are not regular members of a household, such as those who do not work locally. There is probably a slight underestimate of HIV prevalence obtained in national surveys and an overestimate in those involving pregnant women, except in South Africa.

To estimate the prevalence of HIV in concentrated epidemics in high-risk groups one must undertake surveys not only in antenatal clinics, but especially in the highest risk populations, such as men who have sex with men, injecting drug users, and mobile populations, depending on the specific context and country. When dealing with concentrated epidemics methods for estimation are even more problematical. Indeed, to estimate infection rate in these high-risk groups one needs first to know their number at the national level. Establishing estimates of the number of people engaged in such behavior implies working with the populations in question. Many societies condemn and even punish behavior such as illicit drug use, homosexuality, and prostitution. Because of this, people at the highest risk for HIV may be ignored by official epidemiological surveys. If the evolution of high-risk behavior and the number of infections in such groups is not monitored, the inevitable consequence is that efforts to control an epidemic will be inadequate. Most countries have made considerable progress in HIV surveillance in the last fifteen years but there remain areas where it is difficult to obtain reliable estimates of the extent of the epidemic. Population migration dynamics are important in some parts of the world: sometimes mainly internal, sometimes external, masculine or feminine, they can influence estimates of prevalence. Sometimes problems of epidemiological surveillance are political: the problem may be simply ignored, as was the case in China before 2005. It was difficult to obtain information, especially in certain provinces like Hunan where a major part of the adult population of whole villages was contaminated by blood transfusions. The situation has changed since 2005 thanks to greater openness by the central authorities. Other countries present other problems: for example the Democratic Republic of the Congo is an enormous country of which half has no proper roads and where the health services often cannot even perform HIV antibody tests for diagnostic purposes in sick patients. Furthermore in countries like the Congo, Sudan, Afghanistan, or Somalia political instability, insecurity, and war are major obstacles to surveillance of infectious diseases, including AIDS. In most of these cases a large part of differences in data is not a deliberate intention to hide results but simply that the data are just not available.

THE DIVERSIFICATION OF EPIDEMICS

When considering AIDS, it is more correct to speak of HIV *epidemics* rather than a *single* epidemic. HIV has become *endemic* in most countries and is seen in different forms within a country, a region, or a continent. Worldwide inequality of infection is obvious. Half of humanity lives in Asia and yet there is less infection (approximately five million people HIV-positive out of a population of over four billion) than in sub-Saharan Africa (almost twenty-five million infected in 2013 out of a population of around one billion). Even in Africa the variation between countries has increased over the years. In the 1980s South Africa hardly recognized the existence of AIDS and the government did not want to believe in an epidemic.[8] It was not just a political denial. HIV prevalence in pregnant women was still less than 1 percent in 1990 and 2.7 percent in 1992. KwaZulu-Natal province was the most affected at 5 percent. In 1996, two years after the end of apartheid was marked by an extraordinary mobility as townships disappeared, the epidemic jumped to 14 percent prevalence in the adult population. In West Africa, in Senegal, Mali, or Niger, the infection rate is lower than in Washington DC or New York City. Ivory Coast used to be the most affected country, as until recently it had a high offer of employment with, in the capital Abidjan, an excess of men over women. Abidjan was a commercial center for the whole region and money circulated freely.

> When considering AIDS, it is more correct to speak of HIV *epidemics* rather
> than a *single* epidemic. HIV has become *endemic* in most countries and is
> seen in different forms within a country, a region, or a continent.

A sex industry emerged with some ten thousand employees in 1990. Today Nigeria has the highest prevalence in the region with 3.1 percent of adults infected, and with as many as 3.5 million people living with HIV.

In Africa we see enormous variation, and the situation is still evolving. In some countries, like Rwanda, HIV prevalence is much lower than fifteen years ago. In Southern Africa there is a gradual decline in most, but not all, countries. In Uganda there has been a recent increase in incidence, with over one hundred twenty thousand newly infected people in 2013, nearly as many as at the peak of the epidemic, though a population growth of over 3 percent per year has undoubtedly contributed to this reversal of what was the first successful AIDS response in Africa. A further recent development is recognition of the spread of HIV among men who have sex with men wherever this issue was investigated in sub-Saharan Africa. As earlier in Western countries, AIDS has played a role in gay communities coming out against a background of severe societal homophobia and hostile governments. Whereas HIV infection among men who have sex with men may have been underestimated and under researched, injecting drug use seems new in sub-Saharan Africa. As elsewhere in the world, infection is spreading rapidly among injecting drug users. While some governments have been responsive, for example with the establishment of methadone clinics in Tanzania, most are denying the problem. North Africa and the Middle East have the lowest infection rates in the world. The societal context is different, with strict social control over sexuality, and male circumcision is the norm.

Mortality due to AIDS has varied over time, depending on the country or region, due to several factors: the duration of the epidemic, its peak years, and above all efforts to accelerate antiretroviral treatment. This is illustrated by the number of deaths per region over twenty years (figure 1.2). There is a difference between the natural evolution of the

A

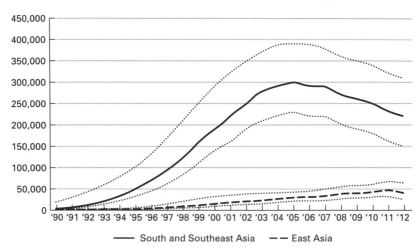

'90 '91 '92 '93 '94 '95 '96 '97 '98 '99 '00 '01 '02 '03 '04 '05 '06 '07 '08 '09 '10 '11 '12

——— South and Southeast Asia　　— — East Asia

B

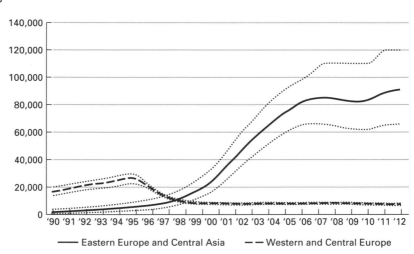

'90 '91 '92 '93 '94 '95 '96 '97 '98 '99 '00 '01 '02 '03 '04 '05 '06 '07 '08 '09 '10 '11 '12

——— Eastern Europe and Central Asia　　— — Western and Central Europe

FIGURE 1.2 Number of AIDS-related deaths by year and region, 1990–2012: (A) South, Southeast, and East Asia; (B) Europe and Central Asia; (C) Latin and North America; (D) Sub-Saharan Africa; (E) Caribbean.

SOURCE: UNAIDS.

C

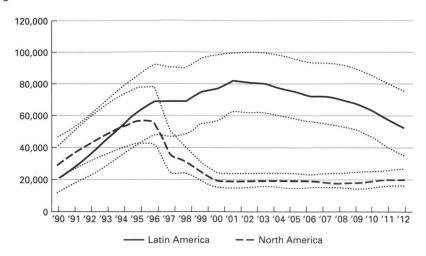

Latin America — — North America

D

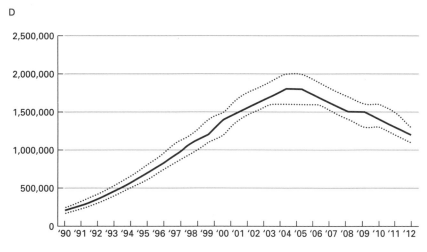

E

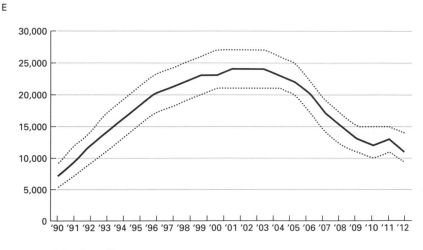

FIGURE 1.2 (Continued)

epidemic with and without treatment, as shown by the evolution in high-income countries. South America introduced large-scale antiretroviral treatment earlier than other developing regions. In 1997, a year after the discovery of effective antiretroviral treatment, Brazil was the first developing country to offer it to all infected patients who needed it. The increase in the number of deaths was significantly slowed. In Africa, on the other hand, the death rate only began to drop around 2005 because of the slow introduction of antiretrovirals. Asia has the two most populous countries in the world, China and India, with around 2.5 billion inhabitants in total. HIV prevalence is low, less than 0.1 percent in China and 0.4 percent in India. However, both countries have major epidemics in some provinces and, as the population is so large, even low prevalence means large numbers of infections. In China two provinces are particularly affected, for different reasons. In the 1980s and 1990s in the central province of Hunan almost one hundred thousand people were infected through criminal blood collection. Merchants connected to commercial blood product suppliers collected blood for a nominal sum from poor peasants trying to supplement their miserable agricultural income. By a primitive system of plasmaphoresis, plasma from different donors was mixed in the same recipient and part of the blood reinjected, thus infecting thousands of people in a short time. In the southern province of Yunnan injecting heroin from nearby Burma (Myanmar) is the main cause of HIV spread. A third wave of HIV is now slowly spreading in the large, economically rich coastal towns, known by the three Ms: *mobile men with money,* as well as among emerging gay communities. New wealth helped HIV soar in China, and also in Vietnam. AIDS is not always connected to poverty: it may relate to fast development, with its inequalities and loss of sexual cultural heritage.

India shows different features. In southern districts with an average of two million inhabitants, infection rates are low compared with Africa, but may affect 3 percent of the population. Two quite separate epidemics are developing. One, around Mumbai and in the states of Karnataka, Tamil Nadu, and Andhra Pradesh, is due to heterosexual transmission related to commercial sex and homosexual contacts. Another, in the northeast, is mainly connected to injecting drug use, again largely with heroin coming

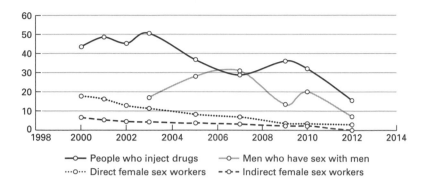

FIGURE 1.3 Trends in HIV prevalence for populations at risk, Thailand. "Direct" sex workers include those who are brothel-based or work in a commercial sexual establishment. "Indirect" means sex workers at establishments where sexual services are hidden by entertainment activities, such as karaoke, massage, and restaurants.

DATA FROM HIV SENTINEL SURVEILLANCE,
UNGASS COUNTRY PROGRESS REPORTS 2008, 2010, AND 2012.

from Burma, but also with Spasmo-Proxyvon, an over-the-counter anti-spasmodic drug for intestinal colic, which rapidly destroys veins.

In Southeast Asia three countries, Cambodia, Burma, and Thailand, have generalized epidemics, with 1 to 2 percent prevalence among pregnant women. National preventive programs have led to a fall in prevalence in the general population and sex workers in the commercial sex trade businesses. However, in the main urban centers injecting drug users and male homosexuals experience a persistent high prevalence, as seen in Thailand (figure 1.3).

In Eastern Europe and Central Asia the number of people with HIV almost doubled between 2000 and 2011, with an estimated one million cases in Russia, and two hundred thirty thousand in Ukraine. Russia and Ukraine account for almost 90 percent of reported new infections, with a 50 percent increase in new infections in Russia between 2006 and 2011, from forty thousand to sixty thousand. Little or nothing is done to stem new infections in drug users, who form the main affected population. National prevention programs, in particular needle exchange and substitution therapy, are highly defective for political and ideological reasons. A remarkable feature is the young age of infected people: more than 80 percent of seropositive persons in Eastern Europe are less than thirty years old, whereas in North America and Western Europe they represent only 30 percent. In Ukraine sexual transmission is becoming more frequent, especially among injecting drug users and their partners. Several Central Asian countries, notably Kazakhstan, Kirghizstan, and Uzbekistan, have recently reported increasing HIV, mostly in drug users. Indeed, Central Asia is at the crossroads of the major drug trafficking routes between east and west.

In Europe general access to antiretrovirals has led to a fall in AIDS mortality. For example, in Switzerland treatment has had a major impact on mortality. Since antiretrovirals have been on the market mortality has fallen to less than one hundred deaths per year. On the other hand the rate of new infection has not followed this trend, even if in 2009 newly declared cases of HIV fell some 17 percent, coinciding with a new campaign of prevention. In France in 2009 some one hundred fifty thousand people had HIV. The proportion of recently acquired adult infections among newly diagnosed people was 30 percent. As in other European countries since 2003 there is a disturbing rise of new infections among gay men. Thus in 2009 a survey among homosexual men frequenting fourteen gay establishments in Paris (saunas, backrooms, and bars) revealed an HIV prevalence of 18 percent, 20 percent of whom were unaware of their infection. Sexual activity and high-risk behavior were rife. In the United Kingdom in 2011 ninety-six thousand people were living with HIV, of whom 43 percent were men having sex with men. A quarter of the HIV-positive were unaware of it, a proportion that has hardly evolved for a decade. In 2009 more than six thousand new cases were diagnosed, a figure that has declined over four years due to fewer cases coming from sub-Saharan Africa. On the other hand two thousand eight hundred new cases in homosexual men indicate a persistent trend toward high-risk behavior since 1999, with five new infections per day among gay men in London alone.

In the United States the HIV epidemic has also evolved (figure 1.4). Thus whereas initially it overwhelmingly affected white gay men, it is now far more diverse in terms of populations at risk. Whereas men

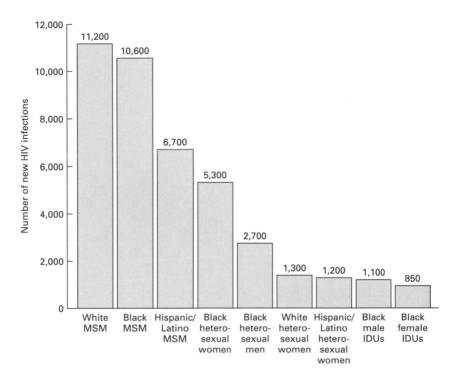

FIGURE 1.4 Estimated new HIV infections in the United States, 2010, for the most affected subpopulations. Subpopulations representing 2 percent or less of the overall U.S. epidemic are not reflected. MSM = men who have sex with men; IDU = injecting drug user.

SOURCE: CENTERS FOR DISEASE CONTROL AND PREVENTION, 2013.

who have sex with men remain the most seriously affected, in particular young African Americans, in 2010 heterosexuals accounted for 25 percent of new infections, and slightly less of all people living with HIV. Women accounted for 20 percent of new infections in 2010, of whom 61 percent were black heterosexual women, a particularly vulnerable group. New infections among injecting drug users have significantly declined since the 1980s. In cities like Washington DC or in parts of New York City, such as the Bronx or Harlem, the prevalence is 3 to 5 percent among men, higher than in the towns of West Africa.[9]

In the United States the HIV epidemic has also evolved. Thus whereas initially it overwhelmingly affected white gay men, it is now far more diverse in terms of populations at risk.

Globally the profile of people with HIV has diversified. For example, in several Asia-Pacific countries, although men continue to account for most cases, the proportion of low-risk women is constantly increasing and has reached more than a third of new infections in Burma, Cambodia, Thailand, and Papua New Guinea. Preventive programs have been very effective, with the promotion of 100 percent condom use for sex workers (figure 1.5). Commercial sex was the source of most infections in the 1990s, but now it is only associated with a minority of new cases.

Similarly, in Uganda and Mozambique half the infections are in low-risk heterosexuals, mostly a partner in a discordant couple (that is, a couple in which one partner is living with HIV). In Kenya and Uganda, around Lake Victoria, fishermen are a very high-risk group and need a special program. In South America, such as in Peru, the situation is totally different: the epidemic concerns principally

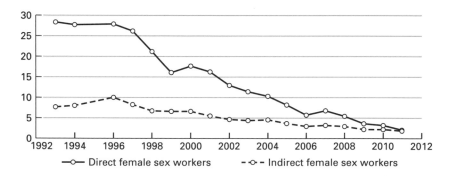

FIGURE 1.5 TRENDS IN HIV PREVALENCE AMONG FEMALE SEX WORKERS IN THAILAND, 1993–2011.

SOURCE: HIV SENTINEL SURVEILLANCE REPORTS, UNGASS COUNTRY PROGRESS REPORTS 2010 AND 2012.

homosexuals. So HIV risk profiles are varied, mixed, and evolving, and we must adapt prevention activities to the local epidemiology, which should be regularly updated, as advocated by UNAIDS with the motto "Know your epidemic."

RISKS AND VULNERABILITY

What determines the spread of a sexually transmitted virus in a population? In their classic work, Robert May and Roy Anderson[10] showed that the reproductive rate (Ro) of an epidemic or an infectious agent in a population depends on three parameters (Ro = βcD) (figure 1.6). First, the probability of transmission (β). For example, influenza is a highly transmissible infection: a person coughing in a bus or shaking hands can infect many people. For HIV the probability of transmission can vary from one in ten to one in one thousand depending on a multitude of biological and behavioral factors. The type of sexual intercourse plays an important role: for homosexual and bisexual men, and heterosexual women, unprotected receptive anal sex with an HIV-positive partner carries the highest risk. Infectivity of HIV also depends on the amount of virus in the blood and bodily secretions—the viral load. High viremia,

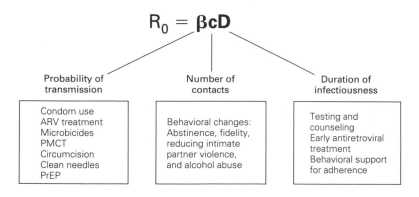

FIGURE 1.6 REPRODUCTIVE RATE EQUATION.

ADAPTED FROM MAY AND ANDERSON (1987).

with high infectivity, is associated with seroconversion or late stages of AIDS. It has also been shown that the probability of transmission from men to women is greater than from women to men. Genital infections increase infectivity, either ulcerative like genital herpes, or nonulcerative such as gonorrhea. Transmission probability also depends on sexual practices and choice of partner and their sexual networks. Studies in Nairobi estimated the risk of HIV transmission between an infected sex worker and her client at 4 to 13 percent when the latter had a sexually transmitted disease. Reducing the risk of transmission can be achieved in a number of ways: condom use, male circumcision, preexposure prophylaxis with antiretroviral drugs for both mother-to-child and sexual transmission, sterile syringes for drug users, and antiretroviral therapy (see chapter 6).

Next is the mean number of sexual contacts with an infected person and the number of sex partners (c). The larger the number of partners and sexual exposures to an infected individual, the higher the risk of acquiring HIV. Interventions to reduce c are all behavioral, such as abstinence, fidelity, and reduction of the number of partners, in particular concomitant partners, as well as structural interventions, such as reducing intimate partner violence and alcohol abuse. Finally comes the mean duration of infection (D). A person infected with HIV can remain in good health for ten, fifteen, or even twenty years. In other infections, like influenza or measles, the mean duration of infectiousness is just a few days. Epidemics such as Ebola virus infection provoke panic, but since the virus kills its host in a week or two, has a nonhuman reservoir, and has low infectivity, this type of infection is rapidly self-limiting—also because control measures are usually rapidly enforced. Key interventions to reduce D include early diagnosis through wide availability of testing and counseling, early antiretroviral treatment, patient support, treatment adherence, accessible and competent health services, and stigma reduction to encourage individuals to access testing and treatment. In mathematical modeling terms, the purpose of infectious disease control is to bring the reproductive rate Ro below one, as it results in the epidemic dying out, since over time less people are newly infected to replace those who died or are cured from the infection. As several mathematical modeling exercises have shown, such a major decline of the HIV epidemic is theoretically possible, though the time span would be much longer than for common infectious diseases. However, many models seem overoptimistic as they often use unrealistic assumptions about user effectiveness of interventions and the long-term coverage of both prevention and treatment. In addition, they appear to ignore the fact that HIV is not evenly distributed in societies, and that Ro will have to be reduced below one in every subpopulation concerned.

An often-raised question is whether differences in the distribution of HIV in the world reflect differences in sexual behavior among countries and cultures. The reply is equivocal, for the relationship between sexual behavior and transmission is complex. If we restrict ourselves to the mean number of sexual partners in a person's lifetime, the highest numbers are found in the United States, followed by Europe: in other words, not in countries with the highest prevalence rates in the world.[11] In addition to the number of sexual exposures, other sexual behaviors and biological factors contribute to the net individual and population-level risk of HIV, such as age at first sexual relations, the number of relations at a given age, age differences between partners, sex with individuals with high-risk behavior, the presence of other sexually transmitted disease, absence of male circumcision, concomitant partners, and condom use.[12]

A key determinant in understanding the spread of HIV is the sex of the individual. A little more than half of people with HIV are female, though in much of sub-Saharan Africa young women aged fifteen to twenty-four are three to five times more likely to be infected than men of their age. This dramatic sex difference is not fully understood. Several explanations have been suggested: a greater biological probability of

---

An often-raised question is whether differences in the distribution of HIV in the world reflect differences in sexual behavior among countries and cultures. The reply is equivocal, for the relationship between sexual behavior and transmission is complex.

sexual transmission from men to women than from women to men, a greater probability that young women will meet an infected partner than the inverse as women tend to have sex with older men, intimate partner violence against women, the vulnerability of the female genital tract to sexually transmitted infections in adolescence, and a higher infection rate of young women by genital herpes, which favors HIV infection.[13] Other differences in sexual culture favor infection. For example, age differences between adolescent girls and their male sex partners are greater in Central and South Africa by eight to ten years than in Europe where the majority of sexual relations in adolescence are between partners of similar ages. In many parts of Africa young women reach the marriage market aged between seventeen and twenty and as a consequence often have sex with or marry older men who have had more risk of infection by HIV. In some populations men may have multiple concomitant relationships with much younger women, resulting in a greater probability to transmit HIV to their primary partners. The range of age differences between partners, the considerable rotation of partners of various matrimonial statuses (divorced, married, single, widowed), and concomitant partnerships all seem important characteristics of sexual networks that explain the dynamics of HIV over and above the mean number of sexual partners. It is therefore the synergy between several behavioral, biological, and social factors that determines the extent of the diffusion of HIV.

CHANGE AND CONTINUITY

During the last thirty years real achievements have been made in the global response to AIDS, as illustrated by a decline in new infections, which globally peaked around the new millennium, and a decrease in deaths, from a peak in 2005 when 2.3 million people died from AIDS, as a result of an unprecedented rise in access to antiretroviral therapy. The sharpest declines in the number of people acquiring HIV infection since 2001 were in sub-Saharan Africa (a drop of almost 40 percent) and the Caribbean (49 percent).

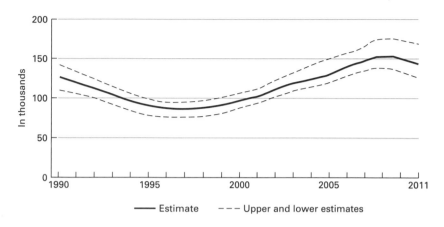

FIGURE 1.7 NUMBER OF PEOPLE NEWLY INFECTED WITH HIV IN UGANDA, 1990–2011.

SOURCE: UGANDA NATIONAL AIDS COMMISSION, 2012.

However, with nearly seven thousand new infections and some five thousand deaths a day, it is difficult to speak of success in the AIDS response. Moreover several regions and countries do not follow the general rule. In Eastern Europe and Central Asia new HIV infections continue to increase, as well as among gay men in numerous high-income countries, despite initial successes in prevention. Finally, the resurgence of HIV infection in Uganda (figure 1.7), documented in 2012 in spite of major efforts at prevention and treatment, should remind us of the fragility of any achievement against HIV, and the need to prepare for a long-term struggle.

2

HYPERENDEMIC HIV IN SOUTHERN AFRICA

———

The Heritage of Apartheid

TRAGEDY IN THE NEW SOUTH AFRICA

Southern Africa is experiencing an exceptionally severe AIDS epidemic, with adult HIV prevalence rates of up to 27.4 percent in 2013 in Swaziland. The region accounts for over one third of all people living with HIV in the world, and the nine countries with the highest prevalence in the world are in Southern Africa. Given these sobering statistics, as well as a continued high spread of HIV, the situation can be characterized as "hyperendemic." Nowhere else in the world is the impact of AIDS on multiple aspects of people's lives and on societies greater.

The thirteenth International AIDS Conference in Durban in 2000 with fifteen thousand participants marked a defining moment in the history of the epidemic. It was the first time that the International AIDS Conference was held in Africa, the worst affected region in the world. It was also the first time that pleas for access to antiretroviral treatment were publicized globally, as a result of street demonstrations by people living with HIV organized by the Treatment Action Campaign (TAC). Furthermore, there was the opening speech in the local cricket stadium by President Mbeki who cited, in a long litany extracted from a WHO report, an extensive list of tropical diseases affecting the region. Then he described the enormous disparities in living conditions between countries of the north and south, concluding that AIDS was a disease of poverty and malnutrition, and not an infection due to a sexually transmitted virus. I spoke just after President Mbeki in what would be one of my most difficult speeches. This is when I called for the international community "to move from the M word to the B word—from millions to billions of dollars to fund the global AIDS response." The president seemed incapable of admitting that AIDS was devastating his people. So he joined other political leaders who were in denial in the 1990s about AIDS in their country, some of them claiming that the epidemic was imported or fabricated—usually by the CIA or some Western laboratory. In 2000, with two million people infected and an adult prevalence of over 20 percent, South Africa was the country most affected by AIDS, making President Mbeki's claims even more unacceptable and tragic. As a result of his views and policies the country became a place for intense debate on the cause of AIDS and on the benefits of antiretroviral treatment, but also of spectacular popular mobilization and resounding legal actions for access to antiretrovirals.

In 2013 Southern Africa included four countries in which the national adult HIV prevalence exceeded 15 percent (figure 2.1).[1] In Swaziland the most recent estimates have 27.4 percent of adults and more than 40 percent of pregnant women were infected with HIV, which represents the highest national prevalence ever recorded in the world. Similar infection rates are recorded in some adjacent provinces of South Africa and Mozambique, where the prevalence in pregnant women was still rising between 2001 and 2011. In contrast, the epidemic is slowly declining in other Southern African countries, such as Botswana, Malawi, and Zambia, but still remains at very high levels.

Zimbabwe is the only country in the region where there are striking falls in prevalence, from 29 percent in 1997 to 15 percent in 2013. How can one explain this decline in a country ravaged by unprecedented political and economic crises? In fact, Zimbabwe was one of the first African countries with strong community-based HIV prevention activities, and the number of new cases decreased progressively from the end of the 1990s, well before the worst of the civil unrest and economic

A

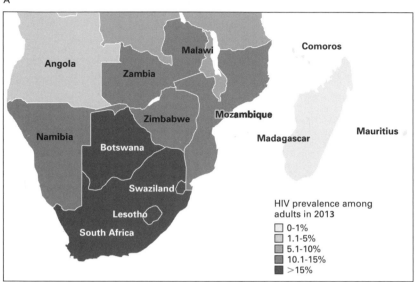

B

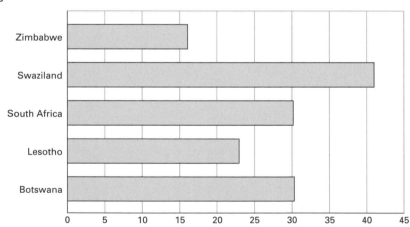

FIGURE 2.1 HIV PREVALENCE IN SOUTHERN AFRICA AMONG (A) ADULTS (2013)
AND (B) PREGNANT WOMEN (2011).

SOURCE: UNAIDS AND UNGASS COUNTRY PROGRESS REPORTS 2012.

decline. This decrease in new infections is at least partly explained by the fact that men under thirty and women under twenty-five have greatly reduced the number of their casual sexual encounters and frequently used condoms during high-risk contacts:[2] almost two hundred million condoms were distributed or sold in 2008 and 2009. These results suggest that intensive programs to change the sexual behavior of young people may be feasible and effective. In addition, economic decline and food shortage inducing massive emigration, and less risky and transactional sex due to dwindling disposable income, may equally have contributed to the decline of HIV spread, which however still remains at a very high level by any standard.

In South Africa, AIDS was first diagnosed in 1983 in Johannesburg. The first recorded infections involved white homosexual men with a rare form of pneumonia, due to *Pneumocystosis carinii*, just as in the United States at that time. In 1990 HIV affected less than 1 percent of the population of South Africa, although it was already widespread in Central and East Africa. Starting in the early 1990s HIV spread explosively in the country, reaching 10.4 percent among pregnant women in 1995, after the fall of apartheid, with continuing very high infection rates. This rapid spread did not affect all provinces equally: there were large differences. In 2009 it was estimated that more than five million South Africans were living with HIV, about 10 percent of the total population and the biggest epidemic in the world, with its toll of deaths, disease, misery, broken families, and millions of orphans. AIDS lowered life expectancy by ten years, from sixty to fifty, and plunged hundreds of thousands of families into poverty and insecurity. More than one third of the miners of Southern Africa under forty were infected with HIV. In a large sugar refinery 26 percent of the employees were infected, each with a mean of six or seven dependents. More recently, the epidemic appears to be stable, but at a very high level: in 2010 prevalence in pregnant women was 38 percent in Durban, 35 percent in Mpumalanga, and 32 percent in Orange Free State. In one community in KwaZulu-Natal, not far from Durban, 40 percent of pregnant women are seropositive, and the new infection rate is still between 5 and 10 percent per year, so that young women who are starting their sexually active life have a 50 percent risk of

In one community in KwaZulu-Natal, not far from Durban, 40 percent of pregnant women are seropositive, and the new infection rate is still between 5 and 10 percent per year, so that young women who are starting their sexually active life have a 50 percent risk of HIV infection after ten years, and death from AIDS ten years after that because treatment is not always available.

HIV infection after ten years, and death from AIDS ten years after that because treatment is not always available. In Cape Town, less affected than the places just mentioned, 16 percent of pregnant women were infected. However, in the Western Cape Province, prevalence among adults was much lower, around 5 percent. When HIV is so highly prevalent, the risk of complacency is real as people may perceive it as a "normal" part of life.

In 2010 alone, close to three hundred thousand South Africans died from AIDS. However, across the subregion, mortality from AIDS has either stabilized, as in South Africa, or declined, as in Botswana, thanks to the expansion of antiretroviral therapy, with Botswana as the pioneer in the region. Today South Africa has the single largest number of people—2.2 million—on antiretroviral treatment in the world (figure 2.2). The increased overall mortality in South Africa since the mid-1990s cannot be attributed to AIDS alone. Other factors have intervened, like an increase in road accidents, violent deaths, and strong demographic growth, but it is striking that in 1997 adult (ages twenty-five to forty-nine) deaths represented 29 percent of the total mortality, and reached 41 percent in 2006 in that age range, which is most affected by HIV infection. Women are particularly affected. Thus, in Johannesburg, the town with the highest population, HIV was the main cause of death in pregnant women according to a recent five-year study in one of the city's largest hospitals. Almost half the maternal deaths between 2003 and 2007 were related to complications of HIV infection, most often tuberculosis and pneumonia.

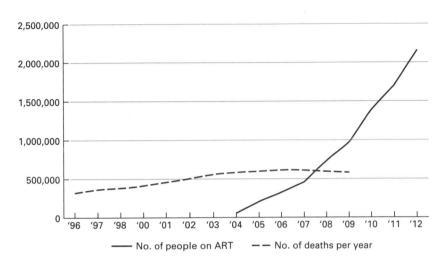

FIGURE 2.2 Number of annual registered deaths per year and number of HIV-infected people under ART in South Africa. ART = antiretroviral treatment.

SOURCE: UNAIDS AND SOUTH AFRICA UNGASS PROGRESS REPORT, 2012.

Life expectancy at birth (the average number of years a person may expect to live if exposed all their life to the same conditions and as determined by mortality in a specific geographic area) is a good indicator of progress and overall quality of life in a country. In both the United States and Western Europe it is now around eighty years, as compared with less than seventy years in 1950. So in sixty years life expectancy at birth increased by more than ten years. In Asia progress is even more spectacular: during the same sixty years life expectancy increased by almost thirty years. Southern Africa was also making progress in life expectancy, reaching over sixty years at the end of the 1980s, but the increased mortality due to AIDS after 1995 reversed the trend back to fifty, the level it was in 1950. In South Africa the higher death rate lowered life expectancy at birth to forty-nine for men and fifty-four for women in 2003 and 2004. Such are the statistics, but beyond the bare figures are the tragedies of millions of lives lost.

The number of children who to lose a father, mother, or both parents has also experienced a phenomenal rise. In South Africa in 2012 it was estimated that 2.5 million children were orphaned due to AIDS; in Zimbabwe, Uganda, and Tanzania there were one million or more, and in the whole of Southern Africa there were fifteen million. This crisis affecting children is one of the most dramatic, but often silent, consequences of the AIDS epidemic in the most affected countries. Many children have to assume adult responsibilities at a very young age, older ones caring for younger ones after their parents' deaths. About 40 percent of children are cared for by grandparents and 30 percent by uncles and aunts. The acute needs of AIDS orphans are housing and food, but their needs go well beyond as they need education, protection, and care until the end of adolescence. We often speak of "vulnerable children" rather than orphans because children whose parents are ill due to HIV are often living in conditions scarcely better than those of children whose parents are dead. In the communities most affected by HIV the extended families with vulnerable children in their care were soon submerged by the double pressure of poverty and illness. Hundreds of child protection committees, often sponsored by local religious and community organizations, and numerous projects for home care gradually provided support to orphans and their host families. However, solidarity is not universal: in very poor regions resources are rare and competition fierce. Discrimination against AIDS orphans, of whom some are themselves infected, is a persistent reality.

Another consequence of a hyperendemic disease is the recrudescence of tuberculosis due to HIV-induced immunodeficiency. It is a major public health problem in South Africa, where half a million new cases were reported in 2009—that is, about one thousand new cases per one hundred thousand inhabitants. More than 60 percent of South African tuberculosis patents were also HIV-positive, and 50 to 80 percent in other Southern African countries. The relative risk from tuberculosis for people living with HIV is between four and twenty times that of those who are HIV-negative. Reported rates for tuberculosis in Africa have doubled since the 1980s and represent some 30 percent of the fourteen million cases known throughout the world according to the WHO global tuberculosis report in 2010. Tuberculosis as an opportunistic infection that is also the major cause of death in AIDS (about

40 percent) in sub-Saharan Africa, and is often the first sign of HIV infection. The two infections together result in considerable costs for health services. To make matters worse, HIV infection has been a major risk determinant for multidrug-resistant (MDR) and extensively drug-resistant (XDR) tuberculosis throughout the world. Such tuberculosis patients are hard or impossible to treat successfully, and cost of treatment is very high. In Tugela Ferry, KwaZulu-Natal, until 2007 6 percent of tuberculosis patients were XDR, all were HIV-positive, and all but one died an average of two weeks after diagnosis. Such patients often became infected in the hospital, and health care workers are at a high risk of acquiring MDR and XDR tuberculosis themselves. Thanks to basic hospital infection control measures, rigorous standardization of treatment, and close monitoring of treatment impact in patients, the rate of MDR and XDR tuberculosis had declined sevenfold by 2012, showing that such a major public health threat can be reversed.

THE VULNERABILITY OF WOMEN

The vulnerability of women to HIV is considerable in Southern Africa, as seen in national surveys. Among fifteen- and nineteen-year-olds, 7 percent of girls in South Africa are already infected, compared to 2.5 percent of boys of the same age—a 2.7 times higher risk for girls. Between the ages of twenty and twenty-four the sex difference is even greater, with four in every five people living with HIV being female. The same differences in prevalence between men and women are also seen in Swaziland and Botswana. As mentioned in chapter 1 we do not fully understand the particular vulnerability of young women, especially as they claim fewer sexual partners than men. It is not necessarily boys of the same age who transmit HIV: in general, older men are more likely to be infected (figure 2.3). The older age of male sex partners implies that women are more likely exposed to men with a higher risk of being HIV-positive.[3] For each year of age difference between sex partners there is also an increase of unprotected sex indicating that with older partners girls or young women cannot insist on the use of condoms. The role

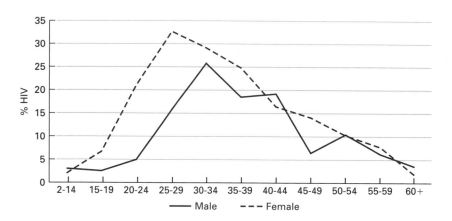

FIGURE 2.3 PERCENTAGE HIV PREVALENCE BY AGE AND SEX, SOUTH AFRICA, 2008.

of sexually transmitted infections as cofactors in HIV transmission has often been evoked, particularly the greater susceptibility of girls associated with genital ulcers. But other factors are more probable, such as the immaturity of the genital tract in adolescent girls, and sexual violence. In surveys of nineteen-year-old girls 10 percent declared that their first sexual intercourse was forced and that for 29 percent it was not consensual. Almost 30 percent were subject to sexual or physical violence by their partner. The difference in HIV infection rates between men and women is also reflected in sex-specific mortality rates, with mortality in young women having increased four times over ten years.

THE DRIVERS OF HYPERENDEMIC HIV

The high HIV prevalence in Southern Africa raises many questions, many still unanswered. The most disturbing enigma is the enormous risk of transmission of the virus at each sexual relation as compared to other parts of the world. These high transmission rates were well documented in several studies on the protective efficacy of vaginal or oral pre-exposure prophylaxis[4] in Southern and East Africa. One hypothesis

> Randomized controlled trials in South Africa, Kenya, and Uganda proved
> that circumcision diminished the risk of acquisition in men by 50 percent.

is that the Southern African HIV strain is a different, more infectious variety. Indeed there is a predominance of genetic subtype C, which might be more infectious or virulent, but it is also found in East Africa, where HIV spread in the general population has not been as dramatic. Its role in an increased probability of transmission will be difficult to ascertain at a population level.

A well-documented risk factor for HIV acquisition during intercourse is the lack of circumcision in men. Epidemiological studies as early as the 1980s in Kenya found that infection in men was associated with a lack of circumcision, but it was not clear whether this was a causal factor or an indicator of another risk determinant, since circumcision is so strongly associated with religion and ethnicity. Randomized controlled trials in South Africa, Kenya, and Uganda proved that circumcision diminished the risk of acquisition in men by 50 percent.[5] Male circumcision does not change the risk of infection of women, who have the same risk of contracting the virus from circumcised or uncircumcised men. The risk is even higher if a woman has sex with a recently circumcised man whose incision is not fully healed. In Southern Africa the circumcision rate is generally low, increasing the overall susceptibility of the male population to HIV, and indirectly of the female population as well. As a result of these findings, large-scale male circumcision programs are now operating in Southern and East Africa. It is interesting to note that in Europe and Asia, except for the Philippines, South Korea, and mainly Muslim states like Pakistan, Bangladesh, and Indonesia, male circumcision is not common, and yet HIV prevalence is generally very low. The reason for the absence of a major heterosexual epidemic in these countries despite the very low rates of male circumcision is not clear, and factors other than the absence of male circumcision must play a role in the intensive spread of HIV in Southern Africa.

Co-infections with *Mycobacterium tuberculosis*, genital *Herpes simplex* (HSV-2), *Plasmodium falciparum* (the cause of malaria), and parasites like helminths have all been suggested to potentially intensify HIV transmission given the association between HIV and other pathogens, possibly caused by lowered immunity or immune stimulation due to chronic infection. However, the geographic distributions in Africa of malaria and helminths do not correspond to the spread of HIV. Epidemiological data suggesting that genital herpes increased threefold the risk of acquiring HIV during sexual intercourse were not confirmed in several randomized intervention trials with acyclovir to control HSV-2 infection. A high prevalence of genital lesions due to chancroid, syphilis, and herpes may still increase transmission and susceptibility to HIV, particularly in connection with concomitant relationships.

Given that HIV is mainly transmitted sexually, what about sexual behavior as an explanation for the epidemic in Southern Africa? When we consider each parameter of sexual behavior separately, such as the number of partners, frequency of commercial sex, and age at first sexual intercourse, studies have shown little difference with other regions of the world. A mathematical model suggested that sexual networks of concurrent partners—sexual contact with several partners in a given time period—considerably increased the risk of HIV transmission.[6] The hypothesis was attractive as the frequency of concurrent partnerships is high in Southern Africa. However, in regions where polygamous unions are common, as in West Africa, HIV prevalence is much lower than in Southern Africa. If we consider polygamous unions as social institutions in which concurrent sexual relations are organized, the simultaneous character of the relations would seem rather a protection against HIV, at least in such closed systems, but not in the context of Southern Africa.[7] Other models have shown that the effect of concurrent partners on the increase in new HIV cases may be strong at the beginning of an epidemic when most new sexual partners are seronegative and that this effect decreased considerably after the peak of the epidemic. In any case, a reduction in concurrent and total number of sex partners should be part of any prevention program.

It is unlikely that there is a single cause for hyperendemic HIV infection in Southern Africa. It seems rather the result of a "perfect storm" of a number of factors that increase the likelihood of transmission, such as commercial sex in a context of poverty, a high number of concurrent partners for men and women before and after marriage, a lack of circumcision, a high divorce and separation rate, sex-based violence, alcohol abuse, untreated genital infections, and large age differences of male and female partners.

It is unlikely that there is a single cause for hyperendemic HIV infection in Southern Africa. It seems rather the result of a "perfect storm" of a number of factors that increase the likelihood of transmission, such as commercial sex in a context of poverty, a high number of concurrent partners for men and women before and after marriage, a lack of circumcision, a high divorce and separation rate, sex-based violence, alcohol abuse, untreated genital infections, and large age differences of male and female partners. Any simple or single explanation fails to capture the complexity of the HIV epidemic in Southern Africa (and elsewhere), and may lead to ineffective prevention programs (see chapter 6).

THE HERITAGE OF APARTHEID

The historic context of the epidemic in Southern Africa, in particular apartheid and its ramifications in neighboring states, has played a determining role in current sexual behavior, and hence the spread of HIV. In contrast to most of sub-Saharan Africa, South Africa was highly urbanized, with some 60 percent of people living in towns at the end of the 1990s, characterized by separate townships controlled by pass laws, with mandatory identity papers for nonwhites since the 1950s. The African countries with very high HIV prevalence all have an important mining sector, with large numbers of miners in South Africa. Although less than in the past, mining for gold, diamonds, or coal still depends on immigration from the whole of Southern Africa. The miners live in crowded hostels according to ethnic or national origin, away from their families for eleven months the duration of their contract. Work conditions have improved, and visits to their families are more frequent, but the still-risky mining environment remains associated with poverty, prostitution, violence, sexually transmitted diseases, and alcoholism. The transactional nature of much of the sexual activity in mining communities is a perfect amplifier of HIV transmission—first among the miners and their sex partners near their place of work, and subsequently to their partners at home. For example, in 1998 in Carletonville—the gold mining heart of South Africa with one hundred thousand miners, of whom 60 percent were immigrants from neighboring provinces or countries—HIV prevalence was 20 percent in adult men and 37 percent in adult women, but 29 percent in miners and 69 percent among sex workers. Another creation of colonial and apartheid regimes were the beer halls for black Africans. Since the 1930s, in Rhodesia, Namibia, or South Africa, the sale of beer was taken over by township councils or mining companies who set up beer halls with a monopoly over the sale of alcohol. In 1958 the Central Beerhall of Johannesburg had thirty thousand to forty thousand customers per day. These venues, and the clandestine cabarets run by the women who made the local beer, soon became brothels around which young women from the countryside lived in great poverty. The explosion of prostitution and sexually transmitted diseases in Southern Africa due to industrial and labor policies and the enormous migration of workers had already been described before the arrival of HIV.[8]

The annual migrations of young men to the mines have affected the population structure of the whole of Southern Africa for decades. For example, in Lesotho 60 percent of adult men are permanently absent from home to work in the mines and industrial plantations. In KwaZulu-Natal men leave the countryside en masse to live in the mining province of Gauteng. Harare in Zimbabwe has twice the number of men than women due to immigrant workers. The migration of young men from the countryside in turn produces a similar migration of young unmarried women who, unable to start a family in their village, move to shanty towns without any livelihood. Several recent studies in rural

South Africa showed that migrating male workers had a higher risk of HIV infection than nonmigrants. Migrants had more casual sex partners and more unprotected sex, and the increased frequency of their return to their community facilitated transmission of the virus to their wives. This circular migration intensified at the end of apartheid, and paradoxically the greater freedom of movement that followed and the multiplication of contacts between previously segregated populations may also have facilitated viral spread. In addition, the combination of a labor system based on disenfranchised men, their segregation, and long-term separation from their families has destroyed marital systems in the whole subregion, with very high rates of separation and divorce.

Sexual violence by men in Southern Africa may also have roots in colonial and apartheid history. More than 25 percent of men questioned in 2009 by the South African Medical Research Council admitted having committed one or several rapes. However, it should be noted that numerous other countries also experience very high levels of sexual violence but without such massive AIDS epidemics. Loss of self-respect due to a long history of domination and exploitation may lead to men who see no other alternative than violence to resolve conflicts.[9] Deprived, disenfranchised, and for a long time without rights, some of these men became violent among themselves and imposed on their women and often their children an exacerbated male domination.[10]

AIDS in Southern Africa demonstrates that the deleterious effects of discriminatory and oppressive societies, like apartheid, can last well beyond their formal abolition. Historic events like conflict and displacement create oppression in hearts and minds and mark families in the deepest spheres of human relations, including in the intimate domain of sexual relations.

THE POLITICS OF DENIAL

In general, progress in the fight against AIDS has been associated with positive political action.[11] On the contrary, bad decisions or none at all have consistently led to increases of HIV infection and death. Southern

> In general, progress in the fight against AIDS has been associated with positive political action. On the contrary, bad decisions or none at all have consistently led to increases of HIV infection and death.

Africa is a dramatic illustration. Take the case of Botswana: mortality began to fall from 2003, to reach the 1996 level again in 2010. This reduction was due to the introduction of antiretrovirals by the government supported by the Bill & Melinda Gates Foundation, Merck, the U.S. government, and, above all, the leadership of President Festus Mogae, who made AIDS a national cause. His leadership saved thousands of lives. AIDS was regularly discussed by the cabinet and Botswana conceived strategies and clear objectives to face the epidemic. With antiretroviral treatment coverage exceeding 85 percent, AIDS deaths fell more than 50 percent between 2003 and 2010. The number of recent orphans has also declined. Although new infections still remain high, they fell by half in the past ten years.

Botswana's ambitious policy of universal access to antiretrovirals, although still late, contrasts that of South Africa, where the impact of AIDS on overall mortality has been overwhelming. Increased mortality was spectacular in women aged fifteen to sixty-four between 1990 and 2000, when mortality was four times higher than in 1985. Such an increase in the death rate of women in peacetime is unique,[12] and AIDS is its major cause. These deaths could have been largely avoided if the South African government under the presidency of Thabo Mbeki had introduced antiretrovirals in the early 2000s. All began well: after the fall of apartheid the new ANC government had launched an ambitious plan against AIDS, and in March 1995 then-Deputy President Mbeki and I, as executive director of UNAIDS, spoke at the International Conference for People Living with HIV/AIDS in Cape Town, calling for mobilization against the epidemic, which raised the hopes for decisive action by the new government. However, at the end of the 1990s, under the influence of denialist American scientists like Peter Duesberg of the University of California at Berkeley, President Mbeki questioned the existence of AIDS, and of HIV as its cause, and blocked access to antiretroviral treatment, which he believed was toxic and could actually cause immunodeficiency. In 2001 a panel of experts convened by the South African president published the *Presidential AIDS Advisory Panel Report* casting further doubt on the efficacy of antiretrovirals and suggesting different approaches for research. The efforts of several world leaders and the discussions that I had with President Mbeki did not make him change his mind. His policies set back the introduction of programs for the prevention of mother-to-child transmission and access to treatment by years. The negative message of the president and his minister of health, Dr. Manto Tshabalala-Msimang, may also have had a considerable impact on the population's perception of AIDS. The minister also sought to influence policies in other Southern African countries—fortunately without much success. In the end the South African government funded the prevention of mother-to-child transmission of HIV and some years later antiretroviral treatment, but only after popular pressure, social mobilization, and legal action by TAC and the AIDS Law Project. Civil society played a key role. The Mbeki government's obstruction of antiretroviral treatment shows that public health policies are not only of academic interest but also have an impact on life and death. Researchers from Harvard University estimated that the delay in introduction of antiretroviral treatment cost the lives of more than three hundred thousand South Africans.[13]

TAC was founded by Zackie Achmat and friends in 1998. Achmat, a gay man living with HIV and an African National Congress militant, refused antiretroviral treatment as long as the government would not make such treatment freely available. The strategy of TAC

Researchers from Harvard University estimated that the delay in introduction of antiretroviral treatment cost the lives of more than three hundred thousand South Africans.

was remarkable: a combination of street action, civil disobedience, the formation of a broad coalition with other sectors of society, and legal action against the South African government. This legal action was possible thanks to the rule of law and the new constitution of South Africa, which forbids discrimination in various forms, and ensures the right to health and protection of children. TAC was the driving force of an unusual coalition consisting notably of representatives from the Chamber of Mines, the Communist Party, trade unions, the Anglican Church, and many scientists. Today, after so many lives lost,[14] and following the impeachment of President Mbeki, President Jacob Zuma's government is pursuing the world's biggest national AIDS treatment program with more than 1.5 million people taking antiretrovirals, over 50 percent of those in clinical need.

PROGRESS AND CHALLENGES

The last few years have been years of hope for the AIDS response in Southern Africa. With the exception of Lesotho and Angola, the annual incidence of HIV among adults in all Southern African countries fell by more than 25 percent between 2001 and 2011. High-risk sexual behavior in men and women has decreased in many communities, including a greater use of condoms. For example, in South Africa condom use for high-risk sex in young men went from 50 to 87 percent between 2002 and 2008. Communication and prevention programs such as South Africa's loveLife program and the Soul City Institute use high-quality entertainment formats (e.g., television, radio, social media) for their messaging and have transformed social ethos. Far from the traditional paternalistic approach to behavior change, these multimedia programs rely on youth and popular culture to encourage low-risk behavior in adolescents. A second major change has been greatly expanding access to antiretroviral treatment, with countries like Botswana, Namibia, Zimbabwe and South Africa now offering higher levels of treatment (figure 2.4). One of the most remarkable developments in South Africa is the emergence of high-quality research on AIDS, public health, and social science in the

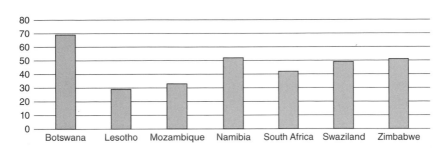

FIGURE 2.4 ESTIMATED PERCENTAGE OF ADULTS (FIFTEEN YEARS AND OLDER) LIVING WITH HIV RECEIVING ANTIRETROVIRAL THERAPY, 2013.

SOURCE: UNAIDS.

subregion—often thanks to new types of international research partnerships. Such centers of excellence should be major assets for addressing a wide range of health issues.

Despite some real achievements the human toll in terms of a persistent high level of new infections and deaths remains unacceptably dramatic. In addition, it will take decades to repair the damage caused by AIDS, from lost generations and orphans to economic loss and destabilization of the fabric of society. A truly exceptional effort by society as a whole will be required to reach very low levels of HIV infection and for the region to realize its full potential.

3

AIDS AS AN INTERNATIONAL
POLITICAL ISSUE

AIDS has been about politics from the beginning. Politics in its original and noble sense: not party politics but that of societal choices, debates, and engagement in the AIDS response. This chapter will discuss the transnational dimension of the AIDS response, which was a new development in health, and may be a precursor of other global solidarity movements.

THE FIRST RESPONSES

AIDS is obviously an infectious disease, but since its discovery in 1981 it has been perceived as distinct from other diseases, largely because of its connection with sex and drugs. However, its image is not only a matter of modes of transmission, but also of the fact that the most affected population groups and people living with HIV often suffer discrimination, marginalization, and deep social prejudice. This stigmatization—religious, moral, and social—has a political dimension that can be a major obstacle to an effective AIDS response. On the other hand, the considerable cost of AIDS and its economic impact in the most affected countries have driven governments to act, sometimes under activist pressure.

A Global Public Good

The concept of global public good provides a strong foundation for an international response to AIDS. It can be defined as a resource, a good, or a service of benefit to all, of which the exploitation or preservation can justify collective international action.[1] The United Nations Development Programme (UNDP) identified global public goods in four areas: environment, health, knowledge and information, and peace and security.[2] It gave a strong justification for paying more attention to global public goods:

> We know that the marketplace is the most efficient way of producing private goods. But the market relies on a set of goods that it cannot itself provide: property rights, predictability, safety, nomenclature and so on. These goods often need to be provided by nonmarket or modified market mechanisms.

This concept reminds us that it is in the interests of everyone to act collectively. The interest of an action is not always immediately perceptible but everyone benefits in the long term. Absence of action or individual action for immediate profit can only have negative consequences for all. This is the theoretical basis *a posteriori* for transnational engagement on AIDS, in addition to the danger of worldwide contagion, even if in reality political pressure is often based on moral considerations and human rights. In other words, in the case of the AIDS pandemic, it is in the interest of everyone, anywhere in the world, that the spread of HIV be brought under control, and that people with HIV have access to lifesaving treatment. In addition, thanks to the globalization of information technology and social media, local or personal events can cause instantaneous and inordinate effects in a world where time and distance seem not to count. The financial crisis of 2009 and 2010 is a dramatic example. The "butterfly effect" was meteorologist Edward Lorenz's metaphor about the "sensitive dependence on initial conditions" in chaos theory. A beat of a butterfly's wings in Paris could provoke a storm in New York weeks or days later. A minute variation in an element can be slowly amplified and ultimately produce enormous changes. If applied to human society, behavioral changes that seem insignificant to begin with can trigger large-scale upheavals, such as the new epidemic of HIV.

In the case of the AIDS pandemic, it is in the interest of everyone, anywhere in the world, that the spread of HIV be brought under control, and that people with HIV have access to lifesaving treatment.

A Transnational Issue

It was unprecedented for international aid. Never before had taxpayers' money in high-income countries been used at such a scale for the treatment of a single chronic disease, with the tacit agreement that the financing would continue for decades, since treatment programs are required for a lifetime. This was the only way that antiretroviral treatment programs, a recurrent cost, could be extended from high-income countries to developing ones. It required the establishment of new international institutions such as UNAIDS, the President's Emergency Plan for AIDS Relief (PEPFAR), the Global Fund, and numerous community-based organizations. To that we can add many large and small existing NGOs that became major players in the global AIDS response, such as Médecins sans Frontières (MSF), Partners in Health, Family Health International, Population Services International, and private foundations such as AmFAR, the Bill & Melinda Gates Foundation, the Clinton Foundation, and the Elizabeth Glaser Foundation. Finally the pharmaceutical industry became involved in various ways around the turn of the millennium.

The First International Declarations

In the space of thirty years numerous speeches and declarations on AIDS have called for mobilization, but only a few declarations made any difference. The power of words might seem trivial and it is obvious that a declaration by the UN does not suddenly change the world. Nevertheless, a declaration by a global or regional platform can provide very useful policy arguments for negotiation at the national level. Politics may well be global, but above all they are local; one must therefore always analyze national policy development or advocacy in their historical and

UNAIDS	The Joint United Nations Programme on HIV/AIDS unites the efforts of eleven UN organizations and works closely with global and national partners in the fight against AIDS
The Global Fund to Fight AIDS, Tuberculosis and Malaria	An international financing institution that invests in prevention, treatment, and care for AIDS, tuberculosis, and malaria
Global Business Coalition	A private sector initiative of companies and organizations investing in public health
International HIV/AIDS Alliance	A global partnership of community-based organizations that seek to prevent the spread of HIV and meet the challenges of AIDS
Bill & Melinda Gates Foundation	Private grant-making foundation that supports numerous initiatives in research and development, public health, agriculture, and education
Wellcome Foundation Trust	Global charitable foundation that supports research in biomedical sciences and global health
UNITAID	Global health organization that uses innovative financing to increase funding for treatments and diagnostics for HIV/AIDS, malaria, and tuberculosis in low-income countries.
International Council of AIDS Service Organizations (ICASO)	A resource for people living with HIV to support an HIV movement that contributes to health, human rights, and gender equality
Global Network for and by People Living with HIV (GNP+)	An organization that advocates to improve the quality of life of people living with HIV
International Community of Women Living with HIV/AIDS (ICW)	A network founded by and for women living with HIV to contribute to improving the quality of life for women with HIV/AIDS
RED Campaign	A privately funded initiative based on the sale of goods marked (RED) by companies to support the Global Fund
President's Emergency Plan for AIDS Relief (PEPFAR)	An initiative launched by President Bush to support the fight against AIDS
The Pan Caribbean Partnership against HIV and AIDS (PanCAP)	Regional umbrella organization that brings together national HIV programs with international and regional organizations in the fight against AIDS in the Caribbean

cultural contexts. For example, if you want to influence an agenda in China you do not do it through civil society or the media as in many other countries, but through dialogue with the Communist Party and various government bodies. For years UNAIDS interacted with increasingly higher levels in the government, until in 2005 I gave a speech on AIDS at the Central Party School of the Communist Party of China in Beijing, where senior Party cadres are trained, followed by a meeting with then-Premier Wen Jiabao. The latter events were only possible because of the extensive work through the institutions and building of trust. They resulted in major policy changes, including policy changes on HIV prevention among drug users.

However, adapting to a local context should by no means imply that different messages are given to different audiences, as the credibility of the messenger or organization would rapidly collapse. It is more a matter of how to present issues, choose examples that resonate, address relevant audiences, and use words that are part of the local vocabulary. For example, how does one talk about human rights in a country like Cuba or China without using the words or terms that shut off any further conversation? In my experience it is usually possible to raise controversial issues like homosexuality and harm reduction in drug users, though it does not work in all environments. Solid scientific knowledge is the necessary foundation of any difficult conversation on AIDS, but knowledge of political decision making and its unwritten rules is equally important to exercise any influence in different countries such as China, the United States, India, or South Africa. A cookie cutter approach for all countries has little chance of convincing anyone, and yet is often used in global health advocacy originating in North America or Europe.

At the beginning of the epidemic some declarations marked the short history of HIV. That of Halfdan Mahler, director general of WHO at the time, to the UN General Assembly in 1987, was the first declaration at a top global political level to demand worldwide mobilization against AIDS, and to predict the social and economic impact that AIDS could have. The 1983 Denver Principles on the rights of "people with AIDS" was the first declaration on AIDS, before any governmental ones. The principle of involving people living with HIV was spelled out. This was confirmed at the Paris AIDS Summit of 1994 where the Principle of Greater Involvement of People Living with HIV/AIDS (GIPA) was signed by forty-two countries. The Denver Principles constitute the first documented statement of people living with HIV seeking more respect and involvement. The principles include the refusal to be victims, an appeal against stigmatization and discrimination, responsibility for their own sexual health, and informing their partners of their HIV infection. After the Denver meeting people living with HIV continued to claim not only their rights, but also recognition and appreciation of their roles and responsibilities. An expression of this plea was the creation of organizations in different parts of the world, such as the AIDS Coalition to Unleash Power (ACT UP) in New York and Paris and the Global Network of People Living with HIV (GNP+). However, people living with HIV on the most affected continent, Africa, were largely without a voice until the 1990s, with the AIDS Support Organization (TASO), founded in 1987 in Uganda, being a precursor later followed by numerous associations across the continent.

So the virus conquered the world in about ten years, but an effective global political response and financial mobilization only really intervened twenty years after the first reports of AIDS in 1981.

The Initial Response of the United Nations System

The initial reactions of international organizations to HIV are surprising in retrospect. Halfdan Mahler, director general of WHO, was very disturbed, like many public health and developmental specialists, by the new epidemic that was upsetting plans for "Health for All by the Year 2000" (universal access to primary health care) and for child health by the UN Children's Fund (UNICEF). During a visit to Zambia in 1985 Dr. Mahler even declared that not too much attention should be paid to AIDS. (This is a statement that we still hear from some traditional public health experts). Dr. Mahler, to his great merit, later recognized that he was mistaken. Equally James Grant, executive director of UNICEF, did not include a reference to HIV/AIDS in the otherwise groundbreaking Convention on the Rights of the Child at the UN General Assembly in 1989. He may have done this for two reasons: first, he may not have wanted to involve sexuality in programs devoted to mother and child, and second, it was already known that HIV could be transmitted from mother to child, including through breast milk. UNICEF was deeply engaged in campaigns for promotion of breastfeeding and its major advantages for child health. To cast doubts on breastfeeding and its undeniable benefits was problematic. This reaction was understandable, but may have delayed an effective response to HIV, in particular the prevention of mother-to-child transmission. It is an illustration of the difficulty for large institutions to adapt and react rapidly to new realities. Other examples are international organizations for family planning, such as the UN Population Fund (UNFPA) or the International Planned Parenthood Federation (IPPF), which were very slow to incorporate the fight against AIDS, as they did not want to mix contraception with a sexually transmitted disease.

It was two years after the discovery of AIDS in the United States when WHO convened the first meeting on AIDS. The consultation was held at the WHO Regional Office for Europe in Denmark, as WHO considered that AIDS was a problem in high-income countries only. Nevertheless, in 1985, at the initiative of Fakhry Assaad, director of communicable diseases at WHO, and Jonathan Mann, then-director of Projet SIDA in Kinshasa, Zaire, WHO organized a discrete meeting at the Pasteur Institute in Bangui, Central African Republic. The spread of the epidemic to Africa and the need to act quickly were at last recognized. A clinical definition was agreed for epidemiological surveillance of AIDS in all developing countries without laboratory facilities to detect HIV. It was only in 1987 that WHO launched a Special Programme on AIDS, with Jonathan Mann of the CDC in Atlanta as its first director, who had founded Projet SIDA in Kinshasa in collaboration with Zairean scientists and the Ministry of Health, as well as the National Institutes of Health (NIH) and the Institute of Tropical Medicine in Antwerp. In a few years Jonathan Mann established what would be renamed the Global Programme on AIDS, in the majority of low- and middle-income countries.

The arrival of Hiroshi Nakajima as director general of WHO led to a continuous string of conflicts for power and visibility with Jonathan

Mann. Dr. Nakajima wanted the Global Programme to become an ordinary program, meaning that its activities must pass through regional offices that in turn would control activities within each country. This implied that the central Global Programme would control nothing, neither the programs nor their finances. There were also ideological tensions: Jonathan Mann supported an approach to AIDS based on promotion of human rights whereas Nakajima preferred a much more biomedical approach, based on medication as far as possible: he considered that too much attention was being paid to AIDS. Mann resigned in 1990. His successor Michael Merson, director of WHO's Diarrhoeal Disease Control Programme, took over from him and, after a difficult start, succeeded in developing a rather effective program within the constraints of WHO.

Between 1990 and 1994 donor countries became more and more dissatisfied with WHO and even more so with the bitter conflicts between different UN agencies that led uncoordinated parallel actions on AIDS in developing countries without necessarily respecting national priorities. The main ones involved were UNDP, UNICEF, and the World Bank, but also bilateral cooperation agencies that gave uncoordinated support to national programs. That led to many AIDS needs not being covered at the national level, to duplication of efforts, with conflicts between health ministers who privileged laboratory and clinical services and other sectors more concerned with prevention and communication, as well as sterile conflicts among UN system agencies. Unsuccessful efforts for coordination between UN agencies eventually suggested that no single existing international organization was capable of addressing all the problems posed by the response to AIDS. This led to the creation of the Joint United Nations Programme on HIV/AIDS (UNAIDS) in 1995.

CONCEPTUALIZATION OF AIDS

Over the years different perspectives on the nature of the AIDS epidemic have evolved, sometimes leading to fierce debate over how the response should be organized. This is important, as a thorough understanding of

> AIDS is in the first place an infectious disease caused by a virus, HIV. To control an infectious disease without an effective treatment or vaccine—as was the case for HIV/AIDS for many years—public health has often vacillated between several approaches and used quarantine, improvement of access to health care, identification of high-risk groups, and epidemiological surveillance.

any health issue is required to guide a meaningful and effective response, in addition to the development of treatment and prevention tools. AIDS has led the way to sharpen our thinking about health, disease, and society in general.

AIDS as a Communicable Disease

AIDS is in the first place an infectious disease caused by a virus, HIV. To control an infectious disease without an effective treatment or vaccine—as was the case for HIV/AIDS for many years—public health has often vacillated between several approaches and used quarantine, improvement of access to health care, identification of high-risk groups, and epidemiological surveillance. The first official reactions to the AIDS epidemic were sometimes rejection of those groups thought to be the carriers of the virus, compulsory HIV testing, quarantine of those infected, closing borders to people living with HIV or limiting the length of their stay, or penalizing high-risk behavior. For example, in Cuba and Bangladesh HIV-positive individuals were initially quarantined. At one point, officials in Bavaria in Germany recommended compulsory testing of anyone in whom the suspicion of carrying HIV could not be excluded, such as sex workers or injecting drug users, but it was never enforced. Swedish law obliged anyone who thought he or she may have a disease that threatened society, such as AIDS, to be tested and, if infected, to be isolated. Access to certain employment or activities was restricted or subject to compulsory testing: Austria required sex workers to be tested every three months and Belgium required it of certain military personnel or African candidates for scholarships. The United States (until 2010) and many other countries restricted entry to their territory for people living with HIV. Today there are still at least forty-five countries that continue to deport, detain, or refuse entry to HIV-positive people, such as Brunei, Egypt, Iraq, Oman, Qatar, the Russian Federation, Sudan, and Yemen.[3]

AIDS as a Human Rights Issue

The new WHO Global Programme on AIDS was strongly opposed from the beginning to any restriction of human rights to control AIDS. Thanks to its visionary first director, Jonathan Mann, promotion of human rights became a foundation of the global response to AIDS. This vision derived from his analysis of the vulnerability of people living with HIV and his conviction that traditional methods such as quarantine and closing borders could not effectively limit the spread of HIV and would represent an even harsher restriction of human rights. The fear of isolation or stigmatization would only force those with HIV into hiding and restrict access to education and counseling for those who needed it most. Furthermore, quarantine cannot be enforced when dealing with millions of people who are living with a virus for decades.

Personally faced with an epidemic of plague in the southwestern United States and then the spread of HIV in Zaire, Jonathan Mann soon understood the overwhelming importance of social and cultural determinants of these epidemics.

> The core of public health knowledge is not only that a blend of individual and societal factors are involved in determining health and associated behaviors like diet, exercise, tobacco smoking, drug and alcohol use, and sexual behavior. Rather, for many, if not most, people, the societal context weighs heavily, if not overwhelmingly, as a determinant of health status.[4]

He reacted against traditional public health and epidemiology that ignore the social determinants of health and disease and limit their analysis to individual risk factors. Their model for disease prevention was based on a belief in rational choices by an individual conscious of risks, forgetting to take account of the constraints and conditions within which these choices were made.

To reconcile public health and society Mann brought together health and individual rights that, until then, had followed parallel paths.[5] Human rights raised the question of social conditions for welfare and health, such as what governments should ensure for everyone, such as elementary education, social security, access to medical care, housing, and adequate food. This first conceptualization of AIDS based on human rights and ethics marked an important evolution compared with the strictly biomedical approach to the disease that predominated in the 1980s, when HIV infection was above all seen as an acquired immuno-deficiency syndrome.

AIDS as a Challenge to Development

In the early 1990s UNDP suggested that AIDS was first and foremost a human development problem. This approach stemmed to a great extent from criticism of the theories and programs of international develop-ment during the 1980s, which were based on the hypothesis of a close link between national economic growth and the expansion of individual human choices. Many people pleaded the need for an alternative devel-opmental model, like Mahbub ul Haq, the Pakistani economist who formulated the paradigm of human development.[6] Since the 1990s the concept of human development has been systematically applied to major societal themes in the annual Human Development Reports of UNDP. The work of Amartya Sen and others defined human development as a process aiming to expand personal choices and reinforce their human capacity and freedom.

> The basic purpose of development is to enlarge people's choices. In prin-ciple, these choices can be infinite and can change over time. People often value achievements that do not show up at all, or not immediately, in income or growth figures: greater access to knowledge, better nutri-tion and health services, more secure livelihoods, security against crime

and physical violence, satisfying leisure hours, political and cultural freedoms and sense of participation in community activities. The objective of development is to create an enabling environment for people to enjoy long, healthy and creative lives.[7]

The AIDS epidemic in the most affected countries clearly involved and affected "human development," notably life expectancy, education, the role of women in society, economic inequalities, and its economic impact. The major preoccupation of development agencies was that the epidemic might represent a diversion of essential developmental resources in the worst affected countries in Africa. The cost of deaths, treatment, and morbidity lowered productivity, increased poverty, undermined human capital, and might even destabilize the fabric of society. This preoccupation enabled the AIDS response to figure among the UN's Millenium Development Goals (MDGs). These goals have become a driving force of several development agencies and countries.

AIDS as a Problem for Human Security

In international, as in national, politics what count above all are the economy and security. The end of the Cold War stimulated much reflection on "*human security*,"[8] of which the simplest definition might be that individual security must serve as a basis for national security, and national security based on individual security must be the basis for international security. Security can then be seen as a public good fulfilling a strategic need for lasting human development. Japan in particular has been promoting human security as basis for international relations.

This new concept covers security against economic deprivation, the quest for an acceptable quality of life, and a guarantee of fundamental human rights including that of freedom of expression and association. Human security deconstructs the relationships between "security" and "state." As a result human security associates state sovereignty with the duty to protect its citizens. It also informs the unfinished debate on the right to, or duty of, humanitarian intervention that challenged the international community in the early 1990s after the succession of crises in

Cambodia, Somalia, Rwanda, and ex-Yugoslavia (Bosnia and Kosovo). According to Secretary-General Kofi Annan, at the fifty-fifth session of the UN General Assembly in 2000:

> Gross abuses of human rights, the large-scale displacement of civilian populations, international terrorism, the AIDS pandemic, drug and arms trafficking and environmental disasters present a direct threat to human security.

By its very size, the HIV epidemic was often perceived as a problem of human security. AIDS as a classic security problem involving destabilization of armed forces and society, as advocated by some like the United States National Intelligence Council, is less well documented—even if military operations and conflict may increase the risk of HIV spread, as recognized by the UN Security Council in its Resolution 1308 on HIV in peacekeeping operations.[9]

THE AWAKENING OF THE MULTILATERAL SYSTEM AND THE INTERNATIONAL RESPONSE

UNAIDS

In 1995 after several years of debate and innumerable meetings, UNAIDS—officially the Joint United Nations Programme on HIV/AIDS—was created. It was conceived by an informal committee composed of a few governments, a few UN agencies, and a few NGOs. There were many reasons for the creation of a UN agency to deal with a single disease. Some were spelled out eloquently in a report by the UN Economic and Social Council.[10]

> Because of its urgency and magnitude, because of its complex socioeconomic and cultural roots, because of the denial and complacency still surrounding HIV and the hidden or taboo behaviours through which it

spreads, because of the discrimination and human rights violations faced by the people affected, the HIV/AIDS epidemic—more than any other health problem—calls for a special global programme. In short, only a special United Nations system programme is capable of orchestrating a global response to a fast-growing epidemic of a feared and stigmatized disease whose roots and ramifications extend into virtually all aspects of society.

Furthermore, a new understanding of AIDS emerged: a lethal epidemic threatening human development, increasing poverty, and reducing life expectancy. There was the conviction that WHO could not extricate the fight against AIDS from purely medical constraints, when civil society and other sectors needed to address this global problem. The 1994 resolution founding UNAIDS[11] recalls that the new program should "Promote broad-based political and social mobilization to prevent and respond to HIV/AIDS within countries, ensuring that national responses involve a wide range of sectors and institutions" and "Advocate greater political commitment . . . including the mobilization and allocation of adequate resources."

When it was created in 1995 its six "co-sponsors" (WHO, the World Bank, UNICEF, UNFPA, UNESCO, and UNDP) wanted to make UNAIDS a simple coordinator for their AIDS activities. When it became operational in 1996, as the founding executive director, I made it evolve well beyond mere coordination, as I was convinced that coordination only was a recipe for never-ending UN and member state processes with no chance to influence the course of the epidemic and the lives of people affected. The joint program was based on a concept that went beyond AIDS.[12] It was an intergovernmental organization in the political sense with a secretariat in Geneva and offices in the regions most affected by AIDS in some sixty countries. The secretariat concentrated on coordination and questions of policy and strategy; it organized mobilization of resources, including price negotiations of drugs and other essential commodities, and evaluation of programs. This new concept followed an uninterrupted series of political discussions I had with players from all sides about what should be accomplished for AIDS at a time when already at least fifteen million people were infected throughout the world.

The six co-sponsors became eleven over the years: the International Labour Organization joined the program, as did the UN High Commission for Refugees (UNHCR), the World Food Programme, the UN Office on Drugs and Crime, and UN Women. A coordination committee of heads of the various co-sponsoring institutions was created, as well as an autonomous Programme Coordination Board in which for the first time in the UN system NGOs were members, representing civil society, including associations of people living with HIV. UNAIDS soon became a major leader in the global AIDS response, focusing on strategic guidance grounded in science and human rights, and balancing activism with the necessary diplomacy. At the national level several more years would be needed for effective collaboration on AIDS between government sectors, NGOs, and international agencies, and it is probably fair to say that there is still a long way to go for an effective AIDS leadership and response in many countries. Under Michel Sidibe's leadership UNAIDS has been at the forefront of defending the rights of marginalized groups, such as homosexual men in Africa.

National Leadership

The global response to HIV is not an abstract concept of the UN. From the end of the 1980s it was grounded in the experience of several countries, as illustrated by a few stories. For example in Uganda in 1985, just after his takeover of power after years of guerilla warfare, President Museveni was confronted by a devastating AIDS epidemic that affected the army in particular. The end of years of civil war and dictatorship had resulted in a sense of liberation, dynamism, and hope in the country, and increased mobility of people. It was probably the first African country in which people took their fate in their own hands in the face of AIDS. Led by the national AIDS control program, and later the Uganda AIDS Commission, and with international backing from numerous Western countries and WHO, Uganda developed early on a dynamic AIDS response that emphasized a role for civil society, with TASO (The AIDS Support Organisation) becoming the archetype of AIDS community groups in Africa.[13]

However, after remarkable achievements in the 1990s and early 2000s, the epidemic stopped regressing in Uganda with adult HIV prevalence remaining at more than 7 percent. In 2013, 1.6 million people were living with HIV (of a population of 37.5 million) and the number of new infections reached one hundred forty thousand, almost as many as at the peak of the epidemic in the 1990s. This rebound of HIV spread occurred in spite of fairly high coverage of antiretroviral treatment and massive investments by PEPFAR and the Global Fund, perhaps due to growing complacency about AIDS among both the leadership and the population. This reversal may have been driven by the initial successful response, the neglect of HIV prevention as opposed to treatment, the persistence of high-risk sexual behavior, the low use of condoms, or by the demographic growth that has reached the phenomenal rate of some 3 percent per year.

Apart from Senegal (where President Diouf had recruited young scientists and public health experts such as Professors Souleymane M'Boup, Awa Coll Seck, and Dr. Ibrahim N'Doye), Cameroon, and Zambia, African leaders in general initially denied the epidemic. As elsewhere AIDS was for a long time an invisible, fatal infection, masked by diseases such as tuberculosis and diarrhea. However, attitudes slowly changed when in the 1990s mortality from AIDS emerged in the African elite, not only in the military but also among professionals, artists, and politicians. For example, in Zambia between 1990 and 2003 a considerable number of parliamentarians died while in office, nearly all from AIDS, as did a son of then-President Kenneth Kaunda. Combined with a clearer documentation of the impact of the epidemic in their countries, this led to a greater acceptance of AIDS as a national emergency. The number and visibility of AIDS deaths became considerable throughout Eastern, Central, and Southern Africa. Rwanda, Burkina Faso, and Botswana then became some of the most dynamic countries in terms of the AIDS response in the second half of the 1990s.

Across the Atlantic Ocean, after years of military dictatorship, Brazil saw the emergence of a well-organized and energetic civil society movement. AIDS appeared in a cultural context of openness about sexuality, and civil society and government remained in the phase of addressing HIV, unlike in other countries. It was the first low- or middle-income country to offer free antiretroviral treatment as soon as it became available in 1996. In 1999, in the middle of an economic crisis and after devaluing the real, President Fernando Henrique Cardoso did not bow to the demands of the International Monetary Fund (IMF) to cut the public AIDS treatment program. It was a political decision, financially supported by a loan from the World Bank. Since then Brazil has become a leader in AIDS policy with the involvement of government, civil society, and business. Health and AIDS policy, intellectual property protection, and access to medication have become an integral part of Brazil's foreign policy. Most Brazilian ambassadors I have met can talk sensibly about AIDS, generic drugs, or global governance, which are rarely part of the classic baggage of diplomats. Brazil's energetic AIDS response was driven by activism embedded in years of struggle against the dictatorship, a well-organized gay community, a constitution that recognizes the right to health, and a desire to develop a local pharmaceutical industry. This meant taking political risks concerning patents, but all along Brazil generally managed not to contravene international intellectual property agreements. However, gross internal inequalities remain a major challenge. Whereas antiretrovirals are available throughout the country paid for by the federal government, actual medical care is a responsibility of the states and municipalities. As a result, in relatively wealthy Sao Paulo or Rio de Janeiro there is reasonably good access to HIV treatment, but in the poor Nordeste one can easily obtain federal antiretrovirals but not antibiotics to treat opportunistic infections.

In Asia, Thailand was the first country affected by the epidemic. This did not come as a surprise in view of the extent of the sex industry, and may be due to a culture that accepts commercial sex (at least for men). From the early 1990s, faced with an alarming epidemic when it was discovered that 4 percent of young military recruits were HIV-positive, the government adopted a pragmatic approach based on reducing commercial sex and making the sex industry safe through the "100 percent condom" campaign for consistent condom use.

In Asia, Thailand was the first country affected by the epidemic. This did not come as a surprise in view of the extent of the sex industry, and may be due to a culture that accepts commercial sex (at least for men). From the early 1990s, faced with an alarming epidemic when it was discovered that 4 percent of young military recruits were HIV-positive, the government adopted a pragmatic approach based on reducing commercial sex and making the sex industry safe through the "100 percent condom" campaign for consistent condom use. Senator Viravaidya Mechai, a minister of information in the early 1990s, family planning activist, businessman, and opinion leader, was the driving force behind Thailand's innovative AIDS response, together with the Ministry of Health. A vast program of awareness about condoms was organized involving many players such as monks, business people, and teachers, and using creative communication methods. As a result, Thailand succeeded in spectacularly reducing the prevalence of HIV among sex workers, from almost 30 percent in the late 1980s to less than 3 percent in 2010, although prevalence remains high among street-based sex workers (see figure 1.6). Hundreds of thousands of lives were saved. Apart from Cambodia and Vietnam, where commercial sex is just as widespread, the rest of the world has shown little interest in this preventive strategy that is so specific to Thai society: in neighboring Burma HIV prevalence among sex workers was as high as 18 percent in 2009. In contrast to this open policy on the prevention of sexual transmission, successive governments opted for a repressive approach to drug use, instead of harm reduction programs that could have prevented the very high HIV levels among injecting drug users. Programs aimed at men who have sex with men also continue to be insufficient, with continuing high HIV infection rates as a result.

Globalization of the Response and the Awakening of High-Income Countries

For a long time American AIDS activists, and to a lesser extent those in Europe, focused their efforts exclusively on the domestic AIDS situation, as accelerating research on treatment, funding, and nondiscrimination were their top priorities—even if NIH, CDC, and AmFAR already

At the end of the 1990s information about the epidemic and its global nature finally spread through a greater involvement of mainstream media, presenting human tragedies behind the figures, particularly concerning orphans and HIV-positive mothers and their infected babies. Media coverage of the explosion of the epidemic in Africa by the *New York Times*, *USA Today*, the *Washington Post*, and major TV channels had a major impact on American public opinion.

supported research in Africa and Asia. Networks such as the International Council of AIDS Support Organizations (ICASO), GNP+, and the International Community of Women Living with HIV/AIDS (ICW), together with numerous regional and national affiliates, worked relentlessly to put AIDS on the global agenda.

At the end of the 1990s information about the epidemic and its global nature finally spread through a greater involvement of mainstream media, presenting human tragedies behind the figures, particularly concerning orphans and HIV-positive mothers and their infected babies. Media coverage of the explosion of the epidemic in Africa by the *New York Times*, *USA Today*, the *Washington Post*, and major TV channels had a major impact on American public opinion. Several celebrities also joined the global AIDS cause, such as Bono, the Irish singer of U2, and Ronaldo, the Brazilian soccer player. Popular media became engaged, such as MTV Networks International led by Bill Roedy, whose global audience could be up to nine hundred million young people on peak days. In marketing surveys MTV found that AIDS figured among the five most important problems cited by young people. Using music, the Internet, and youth culture, MTV's "Staying Alive" campaigns focused on HIV prevention and AIDS-related discrimination across the world. The Staying Alive Foundation, launched in 2005, provides small grants for prevention and care to young leaders to stimulate positive social change on HIV/AIDS in their communities worldwide.

Business also became involved in the AIDS response in the most affected countries, as the epidemic was affecting their human resource base. Thus, in sub-Saharan Africa, companies such as Standard Chartered Bank, Heineken, Unilever, Volkswagen, and Anglo American developed "AIDS in the workplace" programs to promote prevention and support their employees living with HIV. Later, at the World Economic Forum (WEF) in Davos, major mining and petroleum enterprises became interested in AIDS as they realized its impact on production costs. In 1997 President Nelson Mandela delivered a major speech on AIDS in Davos—the first time that he spoke publicly about the epidemic. His strong message was that if businesses did not get fully engaged in the fight against AIDS, they could forget the development of large parts of Africa. The business world gradually became involved in "AIDS in the workplace" programs, though in most cases fairly timidly. As of 1998, the Global Business Coalition on HIV/AIDS, founded by Richard Sykes, the CEO of Glaxo, and later led by Bill Roedy, president of MTV Networks International, brought together corporations involved in the AIDS response. It expanded greatly when businessman and diplomat Richard Holbrooke became its president, and has now enlarged its remit to include tuberculosis and malaria.

A major event for global health was the creation of the Bill & Melinda Gates Foundation, which began to invest in AIDS and other diseases in 1998. Today it spends $1.5 billion per year on global development programs and eight hundred ninety million dollars per year for global health programs and research, including two hundred twenty million dollars on HIV/AIDS, particularly for the development of a vaccine and other HIV prevention technologies. After long hesitation the World Bank also resolutely joined the struggle against the epidemic under President James Wolfensohn, for the countries in which it invested were being more and more affected. In 2000 its vice president for Africa, Callisto Madavo, launched a five hundred million dollar program of grants, not loans, to African to support their AIDS programs. This was a significant development because for the first time it demonstrated that considerable new finances for AIDS was possible, and it also involved for the first time powerful ministries of finance and other sectors beyond health, basically elevating the AIDS response to a major national development issue.

2000/2001: THE TIPPING POINT

Retrospectively, it seems that the new millennium marked a turning point in the global fight against AIDS, the "tipping point" as Malcolm Gladwell[14] called it. Tireless work on the political front and the search for extra financial resources needed for a change in scale in the fight against AIDS began to bear fruit. Thus, the first session of the UN Security Council of the new millennium, on January 8, 2000, was devoted to AIDS in Africa. Vice President Al Gore exceptionally presided over the Security Council with Secretary-General Kofi Annan at his side. For the first time in its history the Council, whose exclusive focus until then had been on classic security, conflict, and peace, debated a health problem—AIDS. This was a unique opportunity to bring the AIDS issue beyond the health agenda to what really matters in international politics: security. The meeting was made possible through the tenacity of the U.S. ambassador to the UN, Richard Holbrooke, who had to convince his colleagues that the pandemic constituted a new type of security challenge. The formal rationale for putting AIDS on the agenda of the Security Council was that it could affect peacekeeping operations, and for some members had the concept of human security as its theoretical basis. The debate was the first enlargement of the concept of security to include more than an absence of insecurity, or war. The same year the United States National Intelligence Council published a report presenting AIDS as a potential politically destabilizing factor and internal threat in most affected countries. Fortunately, some of their scenarios proved too alarmist, particularly because of exaggerated predictions for the spread of HIV in Asia.

Another result of debates in the Security Council was the adoption of Resolution 1308 in July 2000, basically declaring that there should be no UN peacekeeping operations without HIV prevention. It also encouraged states to develop HIV programs for their military and police.

The reason for Resolution 1308 was the potential impact of HIV infection on armed forces, a group with often high-risk sexual behavior, and the accusations that peacekeeping troops contributed to the introduction of HIV in Cambodia after the fall of the genocidal Khmer Rouge. Peacekeeping troops may come from countries with high HIV prevalence, posted to countries with low prevalence, and vice versa. Risks of HIV infection exist on both sides.

Regional and Global Initiatives

As of 2000 a number of regional initiatives were launched by countries particularly affected by HIV, raising awareness of the need to act in their region. In the 1990s the Caribbean had become the second most affected region in the world. In February 2001 at the annual summit of the Caribbean Community (CARICOM), Prime Ministers Denzil Douglas (St. Kitts and Nevis) and Owen Arthur (Barbados) launched the Pan Caribbean Partnership against HIV/ AIDS (PANCAP), together with Sir George Alleyne of the Pan American Health Organization, Yolanda Simons representing the Caribbean Network of People Living with HIV/ AIDS, and myself on behalf of UNAIDS. PANCAP aims at reinforcing the Caribbean response to AIDS, and has become a model for functional cooperation, supporting efforts of a number of small countries with little domestic capacity and with very mobile populations, thus facilitating a more rational use of limited resources. It has been successful in mobilizing resources, joint negotiations to obtain antiretrovirals at affordable prices, training, promotion of human rights, and reduction of stigmatization of people with HIV.

Another regional meeting proved crucial for the creation of momentum for the AIDS response around the new millennium. In April 2001 President Obasanjo of Nigeria hosted a special summit on AIDS, tuberculosis, and other infectious diseases in Abuja in his capacity as president of the Organization of African Unity (now African Union). One head of state after the other broke the silence on AIDS in their country, and collectively the continent acknowledged that it had an AIDS problem, and committed to take resolute action—though at this stage only on HIV prevention. UN Secretary-General Kofi Annan gave a historic speech on AIDS, presenting a plan covering five headings for action and launching an appeal for cheaper antiretrovirals. Shortly before, UNAIDS and WHO had negotiated major price reductions on antiretrovirals with the pharmaceutical industry. In addition the first Indian generic antiretrovirals arrived on the African market. To realize a large-scale campaign against AIDS, Kofi Annan also appealed for the creation of a "war chest" of seven to ten billion dollars per year. In addition, African leaders also committed to spend 15 percent of their budget on health (actually only a few countries would achieve that target ten years later). Finally, after millions of deaths, this summit committed Africa to tackle the epidemic.

In the meantime to "combat HIV/AIDS, malaria and other diseases" was included as the sixth of the "Millennium Development Goals" adopted by the UN General Assembly in September 2000. This ensured that AIDS became a priority for the development agenda of many countries and agencies.

Following a proposal by Ukraine during the UN Security Council debate on AIDS in Africa in January 2000, and supported by the two regional summits on AIDS in the two most affected regions in June 2001, the UN convened a "General Assembly Special Session on HIV/AIDS" (UNGASS) at its headquarters in New York. Forty-five heads of state and government and a multitude of players from the civil society attended this first ever special session of the General Assembly devoted to a health problem. One hundred eighty-nine member states signed a Declaration of Commitment on HIV/AIDS, which recognized the exceptional character of the epidemic and the need to take action at the highest level in each country, involving all relevant sectors in society, not just the health sector. The declaration provided a road map for the AIDS response, and provided concrete targets to attain before 2015, such as a reduction of new infections among young people, and many other objectives in terms of prevention, care, and treatment. The declaration recognized the importance of human rights in the context of AIDS, with governments agreeing to reduce discrimination and sexual violence. During the Assembly tensions often ran high, particularly around the involvement of civil society, and especially accreditation of gay and lesbian NGOs.

I felt strongly that people affected were essential partners in the response, and it required all the authority of Kofi Annan to avoid debates among government representatives only, as is usually the case at the UN.

What is difficult to understand today, and reflects the hesitations of the time, is that in the final declaration there is no concrete objective on access to antiretroviral treatment. The United States and almost all African, Asian, and European countries were opposed to it, except South America, the Caribbean, France, and Luxembourg. Nor do we see mention of men who have sex with men, injecting drug users, or sex workers in the declaration, as a majority of countries found that to mention these words signified legal and moral acceptance of the practices. An example of the mood of the world's states was a vote on whether the International Gay and Lesbian Human Rights Commission could participate as an *observer* at a peripheral round table. At the proposal of Canada, a vote was held just before the opening ceremony. Their participation was only accepted by a vote or two at a plenary session of the UN! I am not sure that even today the same proposal would be accepted by a majority of UN member states.

The Declaration of Commitment on HIV/AIDS also promised to spend between seven and ten billion dollars on AIDS in low- and middle-income countries by 2005. Highly exceptional for this kind of statement, the international community honored that promise. In 2005 approximately $8.3 billion was spent on AIDS programs in low- and middle-income countries.

Game Changers: The Global Fund and PEPFAR

Combined with a resolution of the Group of Eight (G8) summit in Kyushu-Okinawa, chaired by Japan, one of the results of the Special Session was a call to create a special fund for AIDS, which became the Global Fund to fight AIDS, Tuberculosis and Malaria a year later. Donors, led by the United States, the United Kingdom, Japan, and France objected firmly to the UN managing such a fund out of concerns that existing multilateral institutions were too slow and inefficient to manage an emergency fund. The Global Fund was established as a public-private partnership to finance proposals from affected countries, though in practice the overwhelming majority of income is provided by governments, with the United States and France being the top donors. The Fund is administered by twenty members from governments, NGOs, and business, with UNAIDS, WHO, and the World Bank as nonvoting members. Contrary to UNAIDS, where NGOs have no vote, in the Global Fund board they can vote and so are co-responsible for funding decisions—even if they may not always agree with the decisions of the board. Technical advice and implementation of programs are the responsibility of UN agencies, governments, and local NGOs. Thus, the Global Fund does not get involved in program implementation, but has a strong evaluation mandate. By 2013 the Fund had spent nearly sixteen billion dollars to support HIV interventions, and has had a decisive impact on the three diseases it focuses on, with six million people receiving antiretroviral therapy by the end of 2013 thanks to its support.[15] Its result-based and country-driven funding may be a good model for other multilateral funds.

It was in 2001 that financing of AIDS programs in low- and middle-income countries increased spectacularly. This was also a time when aid budgets in high-income countries were rising, so rising AIDS funding came largely from the extra budgets that became available, and did not have to be taken away from other, equally important development and health causes. However, most bilateral and multilateral developmental agencies were hostile to financing antiretroviral treatment, for one of the unwritten rules of international aid was that high-income countries could not be responsible for lifelong treatment in developing countries. Furthermore, the doom-mongers in public health and development proclaimed loudly and clearly that to supply such complex treatment to millions of people with HIV was impossible, particularly in sub-Saharan Africa, since health services functioned so poorly. So there was a powerful coalition against access to antiretrovirals in low-income countries, and some of the arguments were understandable. However, these institutions and experts were blind to the unprecedented and growing momentum to support access to HIV treatment in the most affected countries, particularly in Africa, where less than 3 percent of patients

> Medication was in the north and the patients in the south. However, limited programs that UNAIDS had launched in 1997 in Uganda and Ivory Coast showed that HIV treatment was possible in Africa, and would help to overcome treatment skepticism.

who needed it actually received lifesaving treatment, and every year millions were dying from this new epidemic. Medication was in the north and the patients in the south. However, limited programs that UNAIDS had launched in 1997 in Uganda and Ivory Coast showed that HIV treatment was possible in Africa, and would help to overcome treatment skepticism,[16] as discussed in chapter 5.

When in his State of the Union speech in 2003 President George W. Bush asked Congress for fifteen billion dollars for PEPFAR, he not only took many by surprise, but also fundamentally changed the global AIDS response by giving it resources commensurate with the magnitude of the task, as well as the political and technical backing of the most powerful nation in the world. His successor President Barack Obama continued this highly successful initiative. By 2013, fifty-two billion dollars were spent through PEPFAR, with 6.7 million people benefiting from antiretroviral treatment thanks to American taxpayers' support.[17] Generating broad bipartisan support in Congress unavoidably led to some initial compromises that were not supportive of evidence-based programs, in particular for needle exchange and for sex workers, and a clause that one third of the budget for HIV prevention should go to sexual abstinence programs. Most restrictions of an ideological nature have now been eliminated. The successive directors Randolf Tobias, Mark Dybul, and Eric Goosby pragmatically navigated PEPFAR through congressional meanders and mine fields. Implementation of PEPFAR programs has been largely by NGOs, especially from the United States, including universities and faith-based organizations. In recent years there is a shift toward implementation by local governmental and NGO actors.

As a result of an unprecedented mobilization at many levels, and the creation of the Global Fund and PEPFAR, funding for the global AIDS response increased from some two hundred million dollars in 1986 to $18.9 billion in 2012, of which low- and middle-income countries financed slightly over half. The "replenishment" conference of the Global Fund at the end of 2013 generated twelve billion dollars for the next three years thanks to renewed leadership from Mark Dybul.

LESSONS FOR OTHER HEALTH PROBLEMS

Why was AIDS for several years the only disease that figured so prominently on the public agenda when there were so many other pressing health concerns in the world? This question is reemerging with the growing awareness of several other major health issues, such as maternal, neonatal, and child health, and chronic diseases and mental health. Programs against tuberculosis and malaria have not managed to stimulate such a global movement, though they have benefited greatly from new visibility and finance through the Global Fund.

The political scientist Jeremy Shiffman threw light on the question in his analysis of political determinants of global initiatives.[18] In the case of AIDS practically all critical factors were present and acted in synergy: the power of the players, intellectual and operational positioning, a unified strategy, and a receptive political context. The recent history of AIDS shows that for social change several conditions are necessary. Both a technical and a political strategy are needed, and it is not enough to show how bad a problem is. When a problem is only presented from a technical angle the chances of broad mobilization are low outside a circle of the initiated, especially if the language used is opaque—as is so often the case with health experts and scientists. For a typical decision maker a problem without a solution is not a problem, and requires further research. Antiretroviral treatment offered this solution for AIDS in the mind of key political leaders, as they could see measurable short-term results in terms of rapidly declining mortality.

> The recent history of AIDS shows that for social change several conditions are necessary. Both a technical and a political strategy are needed, and it is not enough to show how bad a problem is. When a problem is only presented from a technical angle the chances of broad mobilization are low outside a circle of the initiated, especially if the language used is opaque—as is so often the case with health experts and scientists. For a typical decision maker a problem without a solution is not a problem, and requires further research. Antiretroviral treatment offered this solution for AIDS in the mind of key political leaders, as they could see measurable short-term results in terms of rapidly declining mortality.

Finally, influential social movements that are able to put an issue at the top of political agendas are often characterized by a broad coalition going beyond a "pure" core group, with a consensus around a minimal program, simple objectives, and an organizational and political strategy to attain them. Above all, it requires leadership at many levels that is both institutional and daring, and is not discouraged at the first difficulties or objections by the powers that be.

Faced with a major lack of governmental action in many countries in the early years of the epidemic, it was community action, particularly in the gay community, that led the response to AIDS, often together with scientists and public health experts. For example, in the United States and France AIDS activists campaigned early on for more investment in research and access to treatment, even if experimental. AIDS engendered a new type of global social movement that questioned traditional principles of public health, doctor-patient relationships, the role of the state and international institutions, as well as theories about behavior change. This dramatic epidemic forced many to broaden their outlook on the world to tackle the new challenges of globalization that need collective action. After more than thirty years of AIDS response, a key question is how to sustain global and local mobilization over the decades that may be needed to end this epidemic.

4

A NEW TYPE OF TRANSNATIONAL
CIVIL SOCIETY MOVEMENT

Since the fall of the Berlin wall and the major financial crisis, the weakening of states has become a "catch-all" theme.[1] Nations would no longer necessarily be the framework for public action. The economic crisis originating with the banking collapse in the United States has demonstrated the fragility of nations, often powerless to exercise a profound reform of the international financial system. Multinationals, international institutions, towns, regions, and civil society groups have become major actors in social and political life. For many reasons—colonization, maritime commercial exchange, development aid, infectious disease control, and epidemics—aspects of public health have historically been part of discussions among nations. The first intergovernmental organizations dealing with health were created in the nineteenth century to monitor epidemics. Today this is primarily the mandate of WHO. Viruses know no borders and recent epidemics, like H1N1 influenza or SARS, have shown the necessity for a coordinated approach to epidemic control. Globalization increases both cross-border health risks and movements of people, as well as greater involvement of an increasing number of actors in health politics. Cross-border commercial interests may dominate those of public health, as with tobacco-induced deaths or mad cow disease.

The global AIDS response has become emblematic of this evolution. Particularly in the early days of the epidemic community groups, more than governments, often organized the response, especially when working with highly affected communities such as drug users, men who have sex with men, and sex workers. In high-income countries, under the influence of AIDS activists, the relationship between clinicians, researchers, and patients was quickly transformed—people living with HIV were often as well informed as their physician.

In 1983 during the second national conference of people living with AIDS in Denver, gay Americans living with HIV met for the first time at the national level. They published the Denver Principles, considered the birth certificate of global AIDS activism. They refused to be considered victims: "*We are 'People With AIDS.'*" They formed committees and chose representatives. They insisted on being involved in decisions at all levels, participating in conferences on AIDS and sharing their experience. They committed themselves to practicing safer sex. These principles were reaffirmed and broadened eleven years later on World Aids Day, December 1, 1994, in the Paris Declaration for Greater Involvement of People Living with or Affected by HIV/AIDS (GIPA). Forty-two countries recognized that the engagement of people with HIV was essential for effective and ethical responses to the epidemic. They devoted themselves to strengthen and coordinate community organizations and networks of people with HIV and to ensure their involvement in programs to encourage the creation of a favorable social, legal, and political environment.

Activist groups, initially mostly of HIV-positive gay men, gradually acquired competence in both advocacy and research. The pharmaceutical industry had to learn to work with various groups to develop and market new drugs. However, these service and advocacy organizations were not easily accepted by policy makers. At the global level, the role

Activist groups, initially mostly of HIV-positive gay men, gradually acquired competence in both advocacy and research. The pharmaceutical industry had to learn to work with various groups to develop and market new drugs. However, these service and advocacy organizations were not easily accepted by policy makers.

of nonstate actors emerged gradually. The WHO Global Programme on AIDS collaborated with NGOs in defining policies to implement, developing their relations with WHO, and encouraging them to organize themselves worldwide. We had to wait until 1995 for this approach to be institutionalized with five seats of the Programme Coordinating Board of UNAIDS allotted to NGOs—though without voting rights, and after overcoming major opposition from countries such as China, Cuba, and The Netherlands in the Economic and Social Council of the UN. Then in 2002 NGOs and affected communities became full members of the Board of the Global Fund with voting rights, and thus became co-responsible for all its decisions. At the country level, civil society organizations were a mandatory part of the Global Fund's Country Coordination Mechanism. While becoming part of the global and local AIDS governance system as well as recipients of public funding, activist groups and AIDS NGOs struggled to sustain their critical independent role.

THE FUNDAMENTAL ROLE OF CIVIL SOCIETY IN THE AIDS RESPONSE

Without effective treatment until 1996, the AIDS response was obviously based on prevention, particularly for those at highest risk of infection. An essential way to influence high-risk behavior is to work with communities that share such high-risk situations and speak the same language. It is a way to accept the organizational differences of groups and cultures and recognize what Michael Polanyi called tacit knowing,[2] essential for communication beyond standard messages. In Dutch we use the neologism *ervaringsdeskundige*—literally "experience expert"—to designate people who have personally experienced a situation or event. When such expertise is combined with scientific evidence and policy analysis it can be a powerful element of policy making and program implementation. In the 1990s Western gay communities proved this with a spectacular decline in new HIV infections. Unfortunately in recent years there has been a rebound of new HIV infections among gay men, possibly following a major decline in deaths thanks to the widespread coverage of antiretroviral therapy, leading to complacency on safer sex and a decline in public HIV prevention campaigns.

Heterogeneity of Activism

Civil society movements and AIDS activism are very heterogeneous and their involvement in global or national responses is very variable. The taxonomy of thousands of AIDS groups is particularly difficult to establish as their specificities and aims overlap, differentiate, or evolve over time as the organizations mature.

For example, in France, after the death of his partner Michel Foucault, Daniel Defert created AIDES (a composite of AIDE and AIDS) in 1984, the first French organization supporting people with HIV to take action, provide services, and influence policies that concerned them. ACT UP France was formed in 1989, inspired by their colleagues in New York. They targeted media, politicians, and pharmaceutical companies with spectacular actions. Some groups specialized in particular topics, like the Association for Research, Communication, Action and Treatment (Arcat), consisting of professionals such as physicians, social workers, journalists, sociologists, psychologists, and also volunteers. Others concentrated on fundraising, such as Sidaction. In addition there are many local groups representing the interests of specific communities affected by HIV such as ASUD (Auto-Support of Users of Drugs). A similar spectrum of AIDS organizations can be found in many countries.

Since 1982 in the United States AIDS activism has focused on access to treatment, acceleration of research, and combating AIDS-related stigmata and discrimination, in the context of poor access to health care services for large numbers of people. The Gay Men's Health Crisis was founded in San Francisco and New York by gay men at a time when some media were talking about "gay cancer."

Since 1982 in the United States AIDS activism has focused on access to treatment, acceleration of research, and combating AIDS-related stigmata and discrimination, in the context of poor access to health care services for large numbers of people. The Gay Men's Health Crisis was founded in San Francisco and New York by gay men at a time when some media were talking about "gay cancer." They soon found volunteers to manage telephone hotlines, share information, give psychological and legal support, and oppose stigmatization. At a time when President Reagan remained silent about AIDS, it was among the most vocal AIDS support groups. Several activists left the group to join ACT UP, a more overtly political action group, standing up for gay rights, denouncing the prices of HIV-related drugs, and demanding more funding for AIDS research. This group soon became international and acquired great notoriety for its spectacular actions during the days of despair when deaths were counted in thousands in gay communities in major Western cities. Numerous local or ethnically specific organizations were set up as the AIDS epidemic evolved. For example, Project Inform, founded in 1984 in San Francisco by Martin Delaney and people living with HIV, specialized in the education and treatment of thousands of AIDS patients with remarkable efforts to make useful medication quickly available in the United States. The Black AIDS Institute founded by Phil Wilson in Los Angeles focuses on the needs of African Americans, who are disproportionally affected by HIV.

Alongside AIDS-specific organizations some large health and development NGOs eventually became involved in the AIDS struggle, such as Medecins sans Frontières (MSF), Oxfam, or CARE. Some like MSF played a pioneering role in promoting and organizing access to treatment, in negotiations on the price of antiretrovirals, and on intellectual property rights. Numerous religious- and faith-based organizations also became involved in AIDS activities, often concentrating on care, prevention of mother to child transmission of HIV, and orphans. Gradually major companies became involved in AIDS, particularly those operating in highly affected countries in Africa, but also companies such as Levi Strauss in San Francisco. The Global Business Council on HIV/AIDS was launched at the WEF in 1997 by a small and diverse number of companies and UNAIDS, with Richard Sykes, CEO of Glaxo, as the first president, and President Nelson Mandela as its patron. Later Bill Roedy, president of MTV International, and Ambassador Richard Holbrooke expanded the Council further into a Coalition on HIV/AIDS, Tuberculosis and Malaria.

Under the presidency of George W. Bush, American evangelical Christians started playing an important role in ensuring U.S. leadership and the support of Congress for the global AIDS response. For example, evangelical leaders such as Rick Warren of the Saddleback Church in California were influential in President Bush's launch of his Emergency Plan (PEPFAR). At the same time faith-based organizations, which enjoy a growing audience in sub-Saharan Africa, also became implementers of PEPFAR, which put them regularly at odds with globally agreed policies, in particular their objections to homosexuality, sex education, and prostitution. Finally what President Bill Clinton could not accomplish on global AIDS during his presidency, he amply made up through his foundation, particularly by skillfully negotiating the lowest prices of antiretroviral drugs.

In Brazil the gay movement was the basis for AIDS activism, with early close collaboration with the government, in contrast to most other countries. Their struggle was for free treatment for people with HIV and local production of antiretrovirals. The response of Brazilian civil society to AIDS in the 1980s and 1990s should also be seen as part of the return to democracy after twenty years of military dictatorship.[3] It was a period when NGOs on all issues flourished, giving rise in 1988 to a revision of the constitution to better guarantee the participation of civil society, and recognizing health as a constitutional right. The AIDS movement benefited from a broad alliance, including the liberation theology faction of the Catholic Church, gay and feminist movements, and other activists for social and health reform. This powerful movement explains in part that the law guaranteeing universal access to antiretrovirals in Brazil was voted in 1996, a few months after the announcement of their efficacy by David Ho at the Vancouver International AIDS Conference. This policy benefited from political consensus from right to left and was supported by President Fernando Henrique Cardoso

In South Africa the AIDS movement was initially part of the anti-apartheid struggle. However the first ANC government was not as active as it should have been in the face of an exploding HIV epidemic in the 1990s, until President Nelson Mandela addressed the nation on World AIDS Day 1998 near the end of his term. Then events took a dramatic turn in 2000 when President Thabo Mbeki questioned that HIV causes AIDS, as well as the efficacy of antiretroviral drugs.

and his health minister, José Serra, who conducted negotiations with pharmaceutical companies to produce generic antiretrovirals.

In South Africa the AIDS movement was initially part of the anti-apartheid struggle. However the first ANC government was not as active as it should have been in the face of an exploding HIV epidemic in the 1990s, until President Nelson Mandela addressed the nation on World AIDS Day 1998 near the end of his term. Then events took a dramatic turn in 2000 when President Thabo Mbeki questioned that HIV causes AIDS, as well as the efficacy of antiretroviral drugs. The refusal of President Mbeki and his government to offer treatment and prevention of mother-to-child transmission of HIV became a unifying factor for a grand coalition. TAC—the Treatment Action Campaign, founded in 1998 by Zackie Achmat, a gay anti-apartheid activist living with HIV, and his friends—became a mass movement with tens of thousands of active members supported by an improbable coalition including scientists, trade unions, the Communist Party, churches, and even some mining companies. The movement became known abroad after thirty-nine pharmaceutical companies sued President Mandela's government, challenging the government's right to allow generic drugs in the country.

TAC had three broad strategies for action: alliances, street action, and legal action against the state—the last being possible in South Africa, but not in many other countries on the continent.[4] Thus, through a suit of the AIDS Law Project the constitutional court directed the government to provide nevirapine for the prevention of mother-to-child infection with HIV. Its argument was that nonaccess to HIV care was contrary to the right to health of pregnant women and children expressed in the constitution. To counter the government's refusal to import generic fluconazole—a potent drug against deadly fungal infections in people living with HIV—Achmat imported thousands of tablets of generic fluconazole from Thailand, one hundred times cheaper than the price in South Africa. TAC also collaborated with international NGOs, particularly MSF, which was a pioneer in providing antiretroviral treatment in townships near Cape Town.

After its spectacular achievements, the movement today is searching its raison d'être and operational model in a greatly changed HIV and political context. In a sense it is a victim of its success, now that President Zuma's government is providing treatment on a large scale (the country now has the largest number of people on antiretroviral therapy anywhere), and international donors have stopped or decreased supporting AIDS NGOs in South Africa. This quasi-existential crisis may be typical of the life course of any spontaneous mass movement.

In Uganda, just out of a long civil war, civil society was mobilized to reconstruct the nation. In 1987 fifteen people, either living with HIV or close to positive individuals, created TASO, the first community-based support organization in Africa. Its first leader Noerine Kaleeba, a charismatic woman whose husband had died from AIDS, launched the concept of "positive living" with the virus, rather than seeing people living with HIV as passive victims—a great example of turning a catastrophe into positive community development, for which they received the International King Baudouin Prize for Development in 1995. In a few years the organization spread all over Uganda. Her successor, Alex Coutinho, transformed TASO into a large professionally managed organization providing treatment, counseling, and psychological and economic support to tens of thousands in Uganda. They were less political than TAC in South Africa as the AIDS situation was less confrontational in Uganda, but also because in Uganda the legal framework could be more restrictive.

Thailand's AIDS response was resolutely adopted by the government in the early 1990s, originally led energetically by Senator Mechai

Viravaidya, a master communicator who came from the family planning field. The Thai Red Cross played a major supporting role, together with some development NGOs such as the Population and Community Development Association (PDA). The Ministry of Health's "100% Condom Programme" resulted in a major reduction in new HIV infections.

A decade later, in 2004, generalized access to antiretrovirals was ensured by mobilization of community networks of people with HIV[5] following an initial government decision not to include antiretrovirals in its new policy of universal health coverage. During the same period the main producer of generics in Thailand marketed a first-line antiretroviral that cost forty dollars per month instead of six hundred dollars. This price reduction enabled activists with connections with health officials and political leaders to convince the government of the cost effectiveness of generalized access for all those who needed treatment. However, much-needed civil society and government action to address the continuing spread of HIV among men who have sex with men and injecting drug users is falling short.

The great diversity in societal activism is also largely a function of greatly different societal contexts. For example, promoting harm reduction for drug users in Russia with its oppressive climate, or organizing a support group for homosexual men in Africa or the Caribbean in a strongly homophobic environment, are a priori extremely difficult tasks as compared to a program of HIV prevention for heterosexual truck drivers or reduction of mother-to-child transmission of HIV.

AIDS AND GLOBALIZATION

From a historic perspective, AIDS appeared at a time when globalization entered a new economic, cultural, and political phase, with ever-growing integration across nations. A movement was emerging in civil society to address globalization, what Arjun Appadurai called "grassroots globalization."[6] This is not without contradictions. For example, the World Social Forum is both an anti-globalization protest movement and a manifestation of our globalized world. With new communication technologies and social networking, global causes and major cross-cutting concerns have found efficient outlets and mobilization opportunities. Some movements and activist networks have become as globalized as major multinational companies. Thus the AIDS movement may be the first example of a new type of transnational civil society movement without clear leaders or programs, driven by social justice and acting simultaneously globally and in a very agile way thanks to modern communication tools. Some examples of more formal global and regional networks are discussed below, but much of the AIDS movement is not that formally organized, and certainly not hierarchical.

The Global Network of People Living with HIV (GNP+) was launched in 1986, around the time of the creation of a special program on AIDS by WHO, when Dietmar Bolle, a nurse living with HIV, sought a means to empower people with HIV and help them share their personal experiences. At the time, and until 1992, GNP+'s main activity was the organization of international conferences to provide a global forum for empowerment of people living with HIV through sharing experiences to increase awareness, building competence and communication. Today GNP+ is a federation of autonomous, regional, and national networks of people living with HIV worldwide. The International Community of Women Living with HIV/AIDS (ICW) was created later as a response to a lack of support for many women living with HIV, even in societies where women account for the majority of people with HIV, such as in sub-Saharan Africa. In 1991 the International Council of AIDS Service Organizations (ICASO) was created, bringing together numerous actors from around the world. With regional offices, a council, and elections, ICASO is a major network that participates in international and regional AIDS meetings and AIDS governance. Under the leadership of Richard Burzynski it played a determining role in the creation of the Global Fund and later its governance. The Society for Women and AIDS in Africa (SWAA) was formed in 1988 in Harare, Zimbabwe, by African women to increase awareness about AIDS and support families confronted with HIV. It involves thirty-three African countries with national societies, some of which are very active. Since 2001 the Seven Sisters in the Asia-Pacific region are an alliance of seven networks representing key affected populations, such as men who have sex with men, sex workers, drug users, and migrants. These networks have vast experience in programs for vulnerable groups and share their knowledge, develop projects, and obtain financing to respond to the needs of their groups.

In 1988 at the Fourth International Conference on AIDS in Stockholm scientists, clinicians, and other professionals working in the AIDS field created the International AIDS Society (IAS), which has several thousand members (I was its President from 1992 to 1994). It organizes large conferences on AIDS, initially annually and every two years since 1994. The first conference was held in Atlanta in 1985 with two thousand participants, mostly Americans. The AIDS conference in Washington, D.C. in 2012 saw well over twenty thousand participants, indicating the extent of the AIDS "industry." Senior politicians and other leaders often participate in these events, and there is broad media coverage. These conferences have become conventions bringing multiple players in the fight against AIDS together, while other international meetings are organized on more specialized themes, as well as regional and national meetings—probably far too many. African scientists created the Society for AIDS in Africa, and colleagues in Asia the AIDS Society of Asia and the Pacific. Such regional bodies are as critical as the global networks.

Since 1988 World AIDS Day represents a force for mobilization visible all over the world, including in tiny towns where its slogan may be visible throughout the year. Its organizer, the World AIDS Campaign, is a coalition of national, regional, and international civil society groups united in an appeal to governments to honor their commitments toward AIDS with the slogan "Stop AIDS, Keep the Promise." World AIDS Day also reminds the public and the media at least once a year of the importance of the AIDS epidemic, when the state of the epidemic and progress in the response from around the world are widely disseminated by UNAIDS.

The Emergence of Transnational Civil Society Movements

The diverse patchwork of local, national, and international AIDS movements together make up the global AIDS movement, which has emerged as the prototype of a "transnational civil society" movement. They have a number of generic characteristics, which may explain their impact:

(1) *High flexibility and nearly real-time communication*, targeting relevant audiences and creating a feeling of belonging to a cause. This is facilitated by the use of email, text, and Twitter, and social networks like Facebook that allow rapid circulation of short messages.

(2) Strong emphasis on local and global *social justice*, and defense and promotion of human rights.

(3) *Leverage and advocacy* to influence political and social institutions to attain the movement's objectives. For example, a group like Blue Diamond in Nepal helped change laws, and even the constitution, to inscribe rights to people of diverse sexual orientation. In 2009 in Senegal, following international protest by AIDS groups and UNAIDS, a court decision to condemn nine homosexual men to eight years in prison was overturned at appeal.

(4) Holding *governments accountable* for financial and political commitments, so that when declarations or agreements are signed politicians and institutions are confronted with their promises.

(5) *Legal action*, used mainly in Central and South America (Brazil and Venezuela) and in other countries where the constitution mentions the right to health care, as in South Africa.

(6) *Public action and demonstrations* such as those by TAC and ACT UP.

(7) *Very informal structures* with local leaders, but without clear global leaders or formal governance body.

(8) *Alliances* with a broad range of actors.

(9) Highly visible *presence at international and national political platforms*, with requests to address them, such as at the UN General Assembly and International AIDS Conferences.

(10) *A proactive media strategy.*

Themes such as discrimination,[7] and after 2000 universal access to antiretroviral therapy, have been the most inspirational themes for AIDS advocacy groups worldwide. Their pressure contributed largely to putting treatment on the global agenda, including through the 3 by

5 Initiative (three million people treated by 2005) launched by WHO and UNAIDS in 2003. However, it took nearly two decades before activists in the United States joined this global movement, as their main concern was access to treatment at home. Fully financing the Global Fund also became a unifying campaign for the global AIDS movement, and is considered an indicator of commitment to the AIDS response by wealthy countries. Governments signing major declarations on AIDS, like the Abuja declaration by African heads of state or the Declaration of Commitment of the UN General Assembly in 2001 and subsequent reinforcements, are regularly reminded of their promises.

Global Governance

AIDS movements have often succeeded in leveraging decisions of governing bodies and institutions. Thus representatives of NGOs and civil society have become expert diplomats, sometimes better prepared than official country representatives. They manage to lobby the G8, the World Health Assembly, or the UN General Assembly. Fifteen years ago, who would have thought that a gay man or sex worker living with HIV could address the UN General Assembly, from the same famous rostrum used by presidents and prime ministers? UNAIDS, the Global Fund, national AIDS councils, scientific committees, and AIDS conferences now have also firmly adopted civil society representation. In some cases, those normally without a voice can access the highest echelons of state. For example, the first meeting of a group of people living with HIV in Addis Ababa in 2000 enabled them to meet the President of the Republic and the Patriarch of the Ethiopian Coptic Church. Sometimes this involvement is just symbolic, but with experience it may become more genuine. It has brought about a new form of democracy by giving a voice to marginalized, and often illegal, populations such as sex workers, men who have sex with men, and drug users. However, resistance to such involvement by civil society persists among some officials and physicians trying to hang on to power. It remains to be seen whether this involvement by HIV-positive people has really led to more effective programs. However, if there is now a greater culture of monitoring and evaluation of commitments and of AIDS funding, it is in part due to continued pressure from civil society.

As compared to major traditional humanitarian NGOs, these new types of civil society movements have a more single-minded agenda, and are often loosely organized around a few personalities. Such informal networks constantly change in nature, sometimes with a reformist, sometimes with a radical approach. They emphasize people's autonomy and empowerment[8] of communities: the capacity to analyze the situation, define the problems, and solve them. Their ability to react rapidly and propose novel solutions is one of their major assets. On the down side, new activist groups frequently suffer from organizational fragility, sometimes following the loss of a leader. Many organizations are ephemeral, with a limited radius of action, a poor capacity for management often related to insufficient funds, and a lack of transparency in terms of representation. This is an emerging galaxy and its long-term future and impact are uncertain. What is remarkable is the emergence of new forms of national and international governance, global civil society movements, and global health.

The Treaty of Westphalia of 1648 still forms the basis for international relations, with the principles of sovereignty of nation-states, equality among states, respect for treaties, and nonintervention between states. The arrival of AIDS transgressed these principles but obviously did not change the rules of international affairs! With AIDS, humanitarian and public health action, inspired, if not produced from outside, occurred

---

The Treaty of Westphalia of 1648 still forms the basis for international relations, with the principles of sovereignty of nation-states, equality among states, respect for treaties, and nonintervention between states. The arrival of AIDS transgressed these principles but obviously did not change the rules of international affairs! With AIDS, humanitarian and public health action, inspired, if not produced from outside, occurred sometimes against the will of the local government.

sometimes against the will of the local government, such as in South Africa or Russia. We may be entering a new era in which not only the globalization of trade, finance, health risks, and information, but also the globalization of moral causes is influencing international relations. Whereas the state remains the crucial political entity, for reasons of sustainability and equity, it is clear that for specific global issues governments are no longer the sole political center, but rather an important hub in several national and global networks of different strengths, to which civil society now firmly belongs. The global AIDS movement has distinctive characteristics but is not a unique case: the environmental movement comes close in terms of symbolic or effective participation of civil society and activists, as seen at the UN summits on climate change. In any case, action by civil society groups, especially people living with HIV, has been one of the key determinants of the achievements of the global AIDS response. Without such activism it is unlikely that in 2014 over ten million people would be alive thanks to antiretroviral therapy.

5

THE RIGHT TO TREATMENT

From the start of the AIDS epidemic finding an effective treatment, if not a cure, was a priority, given the nearly 100 percent mortality within ten years of infection with HIV. Let us not forget that in the early 1980s there were no effective treatments against viruses on the market, except acyclovir for herpes simplex and, partly, amantadine for influenza. Enormous public and private resources were invested in research for an effective HIV treatment. It shows that fast and well-coordinated efforts can lead to concrete results. Unfortunately the search for a vaccine has not yet been as successful. With the discovery of antiretrovirals we entered the era of treatment of viral infections, with major spinoffs of HIV research such as the development of drugs to cure hepatitis C infection. It is not an exaggeration to compare this breakthrough with the discovery of penicillin that opened the antibiotic age. Indeed it is one of the collateral benefits of AIDS. The absence of treatment proved disastrous, especially in Africa. Life expectancy stopped progressing throughout the African continent between 1990 and 1995. For example, in South Africa life expectancy reached sixty-one years in 1991, but by 2006 had collapsed back to fifty years, the same as it had been in the 1960s.

THE PREHISTORY OF AIDS TREATMENT

Numerous ineffective remedies were proposed up to 1996. For example, French researchers who were experimenting with cyclosporine on AIDS patients announced in 1984 that they had found an AIDS treatment. Alas,

> AIDS provoked an explosion of pseudoscience, medical charlatanism, and "alternative" medicine to which desperate patients turned at a time when there was no effective treatment. Among the hundreds of substances sold shamelessly by merchants of hope, several cases of false medication attained international notoriety.

the patients died shortly after. In a context of international competition this experiment was conducted without informed consent of the patients and without approval by the national ethics committee.

AIDS provoked an explosion of pseudoscience, medical charlatanism, and "alternative" medicine to which desperate patients turned at a time when there was no effective treatment. Among the hundreds of substances sold shamelessly by merchants of hope, several cases of false medication attained international notoriety. In 1987 Dr. Zirimwabagabo Lurhuma in Zaire announced that MM1 (for "Mobutu-Mubarak 1") cured AIDS, which was never proved in a regular clinical trial. His work was financed by the African Development Bank and President Mobutu. A few years later a new drug, Kemron, purportedly developed by a team in Kenya but actually produced in Texas, raised much hope, including in the African American community, until the fraud was revealed. Treatment based on thymus extracts was proposed in Europe. In South Africa, even after antiretroviral therapy was proven to be effective, the minister of health, Manto Tshabalala-Msimang, recommended garlic, olive oil, sweet potatoes, and other vegetables to control the disease, while vigorously opposing the use of nevirapine to prevent mother-to-child transmission of HIV. She also supported German entrepreneur Matthias Rath who was selling vitamins to treat HIV infection. In Madagascar in 2000 Zaranaina Christian claimed to have discovered a treatment for AIDS, a simple disinfectant, and tried it on patients without authorization. In January 2007 the Gambian president, Yahya Jammeh, claimed to have discovered an AIDS cure based on medicinal plants, though benefit to patients was never scientifically proven. So even after the advent of antiretrovirals, charlatanism was rife

HAART fundamentally changed the lives of millions of people living with HIV, as well as how the world perceived AIDS and the epidemic. HIV infection was no longer a death sentence, and there was hope that one day the epidemic could be stopped.

throughout the world, driven by greed or relying on false beliefs as to the etiology of AIDS.

Reports by David Ho, Scott Hammer, Roy Gulick, and others on the effectiveness of highly active antiretroviral therapy (HAART) using three different drugs at the eleventh International AIDS Conference in Vancouver in July 1996 were a true game changer.[1] HAART fundamentally changed the lives of millions of people living with HIV, as well as how the world perceived AIDS and the epidemic. HIV infection was no longer a death sentence, and there was hope that one day the epidemic could be stopped. Since then more than thirty antiretroviral drugs have been marketed. Initially antiretroviral therapy was very complicated for patients: it implied precise timetables with numerous drugs and sophisticated dosage programs. Today the drug regimens are much simpler, with the possibility of one tablet per day combining three drugs.

However, current antiretroviral therapy does not offer a cure. A genuine cure implies the total elimination of HIV from the body, while a "functional" cure means control of the virus even if latent viruses persist in various cells.[2] These cells may constitute a permanent source for virus reactivation if treatment is stopped or initiated late in the infection. There are only a few people in whom HIV has been eliminated and can be considered cured.

1996 TO 2000: LETTING THEM DIE

Since September 1996 antiretrovirals have been available in the United States, Western Europe, and other high-income countries. Six months after the Vancouver announcement the government of Brazil offered free antiretroviral treatment to all citizens who needed it. This political decision was made under pressure from activists and the gay community, but was consistent with the new federal constitution, which includes health among the fundamental rights of citizens. In 1997 thirty-six thousand people already received antiretroviral therapy in Brazil, increasing to one hundred twenty-eight thousand of the six hundred thousand persons living with HIV in 2003. Several other countries in Latin America followed. The impact of these policies was directly measurable in a spectacular decline in AIDS-related mortality.

However, very few people living with HIV in the developing world, in particular in sub-Saharan Africa, had access to antiretroviral therapy, and millions continued to die without any hope for treatment.

DEMONSTRATING THE FEASIBILITY OF ANTIRETROVIRAL TREATMENT IN SUB-SAHARAN AFRICA

In September 1997 UNAIDS launched the HIV Drug Access Initiative with the major objective to demonstrate that antiretroviral treatment was possible in resource-poor environments, while for the first time reducing the price of antiretrovirals. Demonstration projects were set up in Chile, Uganda, Ivory Coast, and Vietnam, as these countries were keen to explore the feasibility of such therapy. Quite a few experts in public health and international development were opposed for reasons of feasibility and cost. In Chile, in a single year, the program was adopted as official policy by the Ministry of Health. In Vietnam discrimination of people with HIV was a major obstacle to access to treatment as sex workers and drug users were sent to reeducation camps. As a result, the Drug Access Initiative never really got off the ground, and retrospectively it was an unfortunate choice.

The energetic Peter Mugyenyi of the Joint Clinical Research Centre in Uganda launched the first antiretroviral treatment in sub-Saharan Africa, and later also pioneered the use of Indian generic medicines in his country. Out of despair with both the escalating number of people dying from AIDS and the reluctance of the National Drug Authority to allow Indian generic antiretrovirals under patent into the country, he personally imported antiretrovirals from India in 2000.[3] Independent evaluations showed that both in Uganda and the Ivory Coast the program was a success, with excellent patient compliance. However, the demand largely exceeded the real possibilities. Thus only four thousand patients originally benefited from the program, which forced physicians to make heartbreaking choices. These first antiretroviral treatment programs in sub-Saharan Africa were followed by the French Red Cross in the Congo. The Drug Access Initiative had reached its main goal—demonstrating that antiretroviral therapy is possible in resource-poor environments—and thereby eliminating a major argument of opponents to access to HIV treatment. Whereas thanks to the initiative, the cost of antiretrovirals fell from twelve thousand to six thousand dollars per person per year for low-income countries, this was still far too high and out of reach for most citizens and governments. However, from a strategic perspective, it was very important to have broken down taboos around differential pricing of antiretrovirals still under patent.

In 1999 MSF launched an Access Campaign for essential medicines with proceeds from the Nobel Peace Prize. MSF claimed that because of patents many drugs were too expensive to be used in poor countries and that new drugs were considerably delayed before being accessible to patients. The organization played a pioneering role in several countries, particularly until Global Fund and PEPFAR funding made large-scale treatment possible in Africa. In 1997 they launched treatment initiatives in Cambodia, Cameroun, Kenya, South Africa, and Thailand—mostly on a fairly limited scale because of financial constraints. Partners in

In spite of these scientific advances, medication was not accessible for the overwhelming majority of patients in developing countries. HIV continued to spread seemingly unhindered across the world, and patients continued to die and babies to be infected, both preventable by antiretroviral drugs. The main reasons were the absence of political will, denial by leaders in the most affected countries, and lack of funding.

Health from Boston introduced antiretroviral treatment in their existing primary care and tuberculosis programs in Haiti as of 2001.

In spite of these scientific advances, medication was not accessible for the overwhelming majority of patients in developing countries. HIV continued to spread seemingly unhindered across the world, and patients continued to die and babies to be infected, both preventable by antiretroviral drugs. The main reasons were the absence of political will, denial by leaders in the most affected countries, and lack of funding. The appeal by French president Jacques Chirac in Abidjan in December 1997 was an exception to this rule of global political inactivity. However, speeches were not followed by funding from France or other donor countries, except Luxembourg. So Bernard Kouchner's International Therapeutic Solidarity Fund only had a limited impact in five African countries because of lack of finance. During this phase of fulminant spread of HIV, wealthy countries were not yet ready to accept the financial burden of patients with high long-term recurrent costs.

THE FIRST PRICE REDUCTIONS

In 1998 twenty-nine of the world's largest pharmaceutical companies, including Glaxo Wellcome, the producer of azidothymidine (AZT), took legal action against the South African government's decision to import low-cost generic drugs and impose price control of medicines, which was illegal under apartheid. A South African law of 1997, aimed at making essential drugs available to the greatest number of patients, had given the minister of health broad powers for parallel importation of generic drugs. The companies estimated that this law violated world trade regulations and intellectual property rights, and was contrary to the South African constitution. You do not need to be a communications or political genius to see that suing Nelson Mandela and the first post-apartheid government to prevent them from offering inexpensive medicines to their people is a bad idea, to say the least. It would unleash an international campaign against the pharmaceutical industry in general. However, the European Union and the Clinton administration supported the pharmaceutical industry, an error that would haunt Vice President Al Gore when he became a presidential candidate. Likewise, the United States challenged Brazil's use of generic antiretrovirals at the World Trade Organization (WTO) in 2001, but dropped the complaint.

In 1997 the TAC found out that one of the antifungal drugs used to treat opportunistic infections related to AIDS, fluconazole, was sold at about twenty-five U.S. cents per capsule in Thailand, whereas it cost sixty times more in South Africa. TAC imported the Thai generic form illegally, and was at the forefront of action against the industry's lawsuit. Ironically for the pharmaceutical companies, what was a concerted attempt to block greatly increased availability of cheaper generic drugs catalyzed the world's attention to issues such as the price of pharmaceuticals in developing countries and the implications of intellectual property protection for access to treatment. Under pressure from the South African government and civil society, supported by a vocal global coalition of organizations such as ACT UP, Oxfam, and MSF, as well as the UN secretary general and UNAIDS, the companies eventually withdrew their complaint in 2001.

In 1999 and 2000 the first generic antiretrovirals arrived on the world market, mainly produced in India by companies such as Cipla and Ranbaxy. This move by the Indian generic industry was part of the emergence of India on the global market. It fundamentally changed access to medicines in low-income countries, in particular sub-Saharan Africa, by introducing generic price competition of drugs still under patent.

2000 TO 2001: THE TURNING POINT

In 2000 and 2001 access to antiretroviral treatment in low- and middle-income countries was still not widely accepted politically, in particular by donor countries. However, there were significant advances toward both major price reductions and specific financing mechanisms. For example, in January 2000, just after the historic session of the UN Security Council on AIDS in Africa, the World Economic Forum took place in Davos, where Gro Harlem Brundtland, director general of WHO, and I met with CEOs of major pharmaceutical laboratories to convince them to lower the price of antiretrovirals for developing countries, but with apparently no success. However, a few months later five laboratories agreed to lower the price of antiretrovirals for low-income countries, as part of the UNAIDS-WHO Accelerating Access Initiative. This led to a decrease in prices of antiretrovirals still under patent to fifteen hundred dollars per person per year. For the first time the UN, through Secretary General Kofi Annan, also became directly involved in price negotiations with major pharmaceutical companies. This spectacular decrease in price and the corresponding increase in number of patients are shown for Uganda in figure 5.1. This price was still much too high for most people in low-income countries, especially in Africa, in spite of the progress it represented.

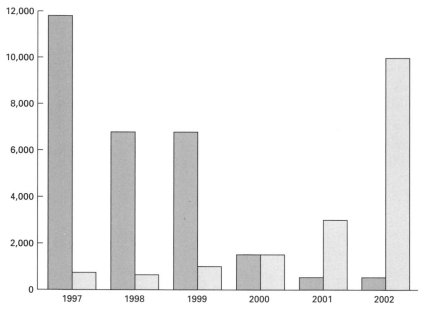

■ Price of first-line regimen in U.S. dollars per year
☐ Number of people treated at end of the year

FIGURE 5.1 TRENDS IN THE COST OF ANTIRETROVIRAL (ARV) DRUGS IN UGANDA COMPARED TO THE NUMBER OF PEOPLE UNDER TREATMENT, 1997–2002.

Lack of specific finance, combined with prices that were still too high, limited the immediate impact of the Accelerating Access Initiative, which generated criticism from various quarters. Among the negative reactions to this initiative ("no good deed goes unpunished") were those of AIDS activists, for whom the agreement did not go far enough and excluded generics, and African health ministers who, led by South Africa, claimed not to have been consulted. The great majority of them remained opposed to the introduction of antiretroviral treatment in their countries, with exceptions such as Senegal, Uganda, Botswana, and Rwanda.

The thirteenth International Conference on AIDS in Durban in 2000 was the occasion to globally publicize the dramatic need for access to HIV treatment. Nelson Mandela made a resounding appeal at the close of the conference, after a disastrous speech by President Thabo Mbeki at the opening ceremony, in which Mbeki stressed that the cause of AIDS was poverty (implying not HIV). There were public demonstrations and huge worldwide media coverage. Participants highlighted the financial obstacles to treatment in the poorest nations, and attacked patents on essential drugs as the cause for their inaccessibility.

In September 2000 the European Commission organized a round table on access to HIV treatment led by its president, Romano Prodi, bringing together for the first time major pharmaceutical laboratories and producers of generics. This was another important step—for the first time all key players were in the same room. At the meeting Yusuf Hamied, CEO of Indian company CIPLA, made the spectacular offer to provide antiretroviral therapy for six hundred to eight hundred dollars per person per year. In February 2001 Dr. Hamied reduced his offer to a then-astonishing three hundred dollars, but contrary to many people's expectations the uptake was very disappointing—mainly due to a lack of a funding mechanism.

Now that generic antiretrovirals were available at affordable prices, it was important to ensure an international legal framework allowing countries to use generic versions of drugs still under patent as part of the Trade-Related Aspects of Intellectual Property Rights (TRIPS) agreement. Pascal Lamy, European commissioner for trade at the time of the

2000 European Commission Round Table on HIV, and then-director general of WTO, played a crucial role in seeking a compromise over the TRIPS agreement, which was adopted by WTO in Doha in 2001. The declaration on the TRIPS agreement and public health stated that TRIPS should not prevent member states from taking measures to protect public health, allowing them to override patent laws for public health emergencies such as AIDS through compulsory licensing and local production, with fair compensation to the patent holder. It also extended the obligation for the "least developed countries" to adopt TRIPS to 2016, which is now looming. The procedures were onerous, and the agreement failed to address the important issue of importation of generics from third-party countries, basically India, but this was solved by a later agreement. However, it constituted yet another building block toward wide access to HIV treatment.

In spite of all this progress international development agencies such as U.S. Agency for International Development (USAID) and the United Kingdom's Department for International Development refused to fund access to antiretroviral treatment. The opposition of wealthy countries, joined by Africa and Asia, resulted in the absence of a goal on access to treatment in the Declaration of Commitment of the UN General Assembly Special Session on HIV/AIDS in June 2001—something that is hard to understand today. Apart from France, Luxembourg, the Caribbean countries, and the South American Rio Group, UN member states were staunchly opposed to the inclusion of such an objective. This rejection was supported by mainstream public health and international development experts and agencies such as the World Bank. They invoked poor cost effectiveness of HIV treatment, as compared to prevention and the control of other diseases of poor populations, as well as the deplorable state of health services in sub-Saharan Africa, which was indeed often the case—then as today. AIDS clearly disrupted plans and orthodoxy in public health and development, and the debate did not shine in terms of scientific rigor. Thus a senior economist at the World Bank wrote in 1998: "The brutal fact" was that "those who could pay for Africa's AIDS therapy—the pharmaceutical industry, by way of price cuts and rich country tax payers, by way of foreign aid—are very unlikely to be

Although differential pricing of pharmaceuticals is not new and has been practiced for developing countries for vaccines, antiretrovirals were the first drugs still under patent for which this was accepted.

persuaded to do so." The administrator of USAID even declared that Africans would not be able to take medication at prescribed times as their notion of time was inaccurate or that they did not wear watches. Only a few years later, the United States would be leading the largest international health effort ever to bring HIV treatment to Africa. It took WHO until 2003 to include antiretrovirals on the list of essential drugs, which many countries follow for their own drug policies.[4]

Although differential pricing of pharmaceuticals is not new and has been practiced for developing countries for vaccines, antiretrovirals were the first drugs still under patent for which this was accepted. In addition, generic competition further decreased prices to their present level of one hundred to two hundred dollars per person per year for low-income countries. As of 2002 the Clinton Foundation's AIDS initiative played a major role in further engaging (mostly Indian) manufacturers of generics, helping them reduce production costs, and brokering bulk purchase of antiretroviral drugs by countries and international institutions to ensure a guaranteed supply at low prices.

TOWARD UNIVERSAL ACCESS

Now that the cost of treatment had declined to affordable levels, money was needed, and a lot:[5] as a start seven billion dollars per year as Kofi Annan had asked in his speech in Abuja in April 2001. Price reductions of drugs only had a large-scale impact when financing mechanisms were ready. After the Special Session on HIV/AIDS at the UN General Assembly and the Japan-hosted G8 summit at Kyushu Okinawa, the Global Fund was created in 2002 with Richard Feachem as first executive director.

The taboo of international funding of lifetime treatment was broken. One year later, President George W. Bush launched PEPFAR, which was initially led by Randalf Tobias, former chief executive of pharmaceutical company Eli Lilly. PEPFAR first concentrated its efforts on the fifteen countries most affected by HIV, with now millions of people owing their daily survival to American taxpayers. Around the same time WHO and UNAIDS launched the audacious 3 × 5 Initiative in 2003, aiming to treat three million people by 2005—an initiative driven by WHO's Jim Kim, now president of the World Bank, and J. W. Lee, WHO's director general.

Some countries did not wait for contributions from the international community. I already mentioned Brazil, but there is also West African Senegal, a pioneer in access to treatment, with Souleymane M'Boup, Ibrahim N'Doye, and Awa Coll-Seck as champions, that launched HIV treatment programs with local funding until external donors joined in. At the southern end of the continent Festus Mogae, president of Botswana, one of the most affected countries in the world, personally launched an ambitious program with support from the Gates Foundation and pharmaceutical company Merck aiming to offer HIV treatment to all citizens. Botswana now has an 85 percent coverage of treatment, with a great decrease in mortality, though new HIV infections continue to be high. This evolution contrasts with what happened in neighboring South Africa where mortality, especially of women, continued to increase because no treatment was provided as a result of the AIDS policies of President Mbeki's government

This long road toward universal access to antiretroviral treatment has been strewn with obstacles. Progress depended on aligning a broad and complex set of forces: a favorable international and domestic political environment and public opinion for a moral cause, a unified strategy by the very diverse AIDS movement, a drastic cut in drug prices with realistic options for both research-based and generic pharmaceutical companies, changed rules of international TRIPS agreements on patents, specific financing mechanisms, delivery capacity on the ground, widely acceptable accountability standards and systems, and more. It all happened thanks to a unique coalition and a favorable economic and political context, and very much driven by the tragedy of millions of

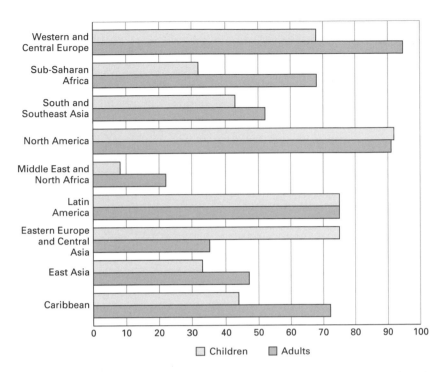

FIGURE 5.2 ESTIMATED PERCENTAGE ANTIRETROVIRAL TREATMENT (ART)
COVERAGE BASED ON WHO 2010 GUIDELINES.

SOURCE: UNAIDS, REPORT ON THE GLOBAL EPIDEMIC, 2013.

deaths with seemingly no end to the epidemic in sight. The final result
is a spectacular increase in people under treatment. Around ten million
are now under treatment in 2013, out of a total of thirty-five million
people living with HIV who at some stage in their life will need antiretroviral therapy.

In addition to persistent low treatment coverage for children (figure 5.2),
men are notably less likely than women worldwide to receive antiretroviral therapy. Gaps in treatment also vary by region, with the largest
treatment gap currently seen in North Africa and the Middle East and
in certain countries, such as the Democratic Republic of the Congo and
Nigeria. Unexpectedly, in sub-Saharan Africa women have better access

to treatment than men. This unusually favorable situation for women may be due to widespread screening for HIV in pregnant women, as an initial step to treatment. As a result of this still-growing coverage, global mortality from HIV infection started to decline as of 2005, when 2.2 million people died, as compared to 1.5 million in 2013.[6]

THE LONG-TERM STAKES OF ANTIRETROVIRAL TREATMENT

Now that antiretroviral treatment is firmly established, other stakes emerge beyond this initial stage. Nelson Mandela once said "that after climbing a great hill, one only finds that there are many more hills to climb." This is certainly true of the still-young history of antiretroviral therapy. Chapters 7 and 9 discuss the crucial problem of long-term finance and the growing difficulty to extend treatment to the ever-increasing number of patients who will need it in the future. In spite of a successful replenishment of the Global Fund in 2013, when twelve billion dollars were raised for three years, international funding for HIV activities has been flattening off. Some of the decline in international funding has been compensated by greater domestic funding in middle-income countries. But there are other crucial technical and operational stakes besides financing.

The first challenge is a technical issue: *when to start treatment* from a perspective of clinical benefit. There is no consensus among clinicians on when to start such treatment, as the benefits and risks are assessed differently by various groups of experts. Thus the U.S. and WHO treatment guidelines recommend the initiation of antiretroviral treatment in either all people living with HIV or with CD4 lymphocyte counts of five hundred per mm³ or below. This is based on convincing evidence

Now that antiretroviral treatment is firmly established, other stakes emerge beyond this initial stage. Nelson Mandela once said "that after climbing a great hill, one only finds that there are many more hills to climb."

about the need to suppress viral replication early in infection to inhibit immune deterioration and disease progression, and the opportunity to reduce transmission to sex partners following viral suppression in the infected individual.[7] In contrast, European and British recommendations are more conservative, reflecting concerns about both clinical and cost effectiveness, and side effects of long-term antiretroviral treatment.[8] Operational and financial implications of the former treatment policy are huge, as it would imply that today over thirty-five million people in the world need antiretroviral treatment.

A second challenge is the use and effectiveness of *antiretroviral treatment to reduce or stop HIV transmission* at the population level. A landmark study called HPTN 052[9] demonstrated that providing antiretroviral treatment to the infected member of a discordant couple reduced the risk of transmission by over 95 percent, and in KwaZulu-Natal and China there is some ecological evidence that antiretroviral treatment has contributed to a decrease in incidence at the population level. In contrast, a study of discordant couples in Uganda found no impact on transmission of treating the infected partner, and incidence remains high among men who have sex with men in numerous Western cities with high rates of HIV testing and coverage of antiretroviral treatment. So the jury is still out on the population-level effectiveness of this approach. Results from major population-based trials in Southern Africa may resolve this important policy question.

Third, *operational challenges* to providing lifelong antiretroviral therapy are formidable anywhere in the world. Thus too many patients present to the health service very late in the course of their HIV infection, when they already have severe immunodeficiency, which makes treatment less effective. Disturbingly, a systematic review of early mortality in adults initiating antiretroviral treatment in low- and middle-income countries in 2011 found a median of one hundred twenty-four CD4 lymphocytes per mm^3 at the start of therapy.[10] As a result, in sub-Saharan Africa between 8 and 26 percent of patients die in the first months of treatment. Data from a clinic at Khayelitsha township,[11] near Cape Town, showed that most patients who presented with a CD4 cell count below fifty cells per mm^3, which indicates an almost complete destruction of the immune system, died even if put on immediate antiretroviral treatment. Less immunodepressed patients had a much better chance of survival.[12]

In England in 2009, of eighty-six thousand five hundred people newly diagnosed as HIV-positive, a quarter was unaware of their infection. More widespread access to testing, particularly for those at highest risk, will be needed to further decrease mortality from HIV infection. Knowing one's infection status is only a first step in a complex cascade required to ensure clinical improvement and immune restoration, as well as suppressing viral excretion.

At each step of the cascade (figure 5.3) compliance may diminish and reduce the overall effectiveness of HIV services. Thus in the United

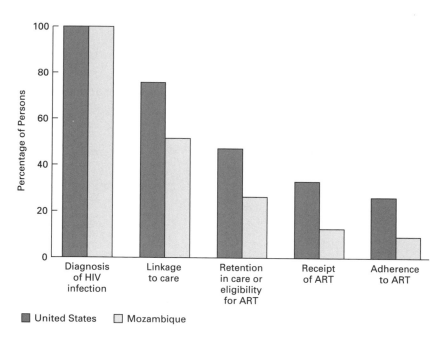

FIGURE 5.3 HIV treatment cascade in the United States and Mozambique from time of diagnosis showing comparative linkage to and retention in care, and receipt and adherence to antiretroviral therapy (ART). From Piot and Quinn 2013, with data from Gardner et al. 2011 and Micek et al. 2009. Data for adherence to ART for the U.S. represent the percentage of individuals virally suppressed, whereas for Mozambique the data were established by questionnaire and pill count because viral levels were not obtained.

States only 28 percent of people diagnosed with HIV infection had undetectable viral levels, with the majority of HIV-positive individuals continuing to be infectious. Similar data for Mozambique are even more sobering. Treatment adherence is a major component of this cascade, and is very unequal across different studies. Whereas one study of twenty-seven thousand individuals in Zambia found that adherence was almost as high as in Europe, other cohort studies in several African countries showed much less favorable results, with worrying mortality figures. After four years of follow-up a UNAIDS report estimated that 70 percent of patients adhered to their treatment in sub-Saharan Africa,[13] ten percentage points less than the mean worldwide.

There are multiple reasons for poor uptake of and adherence to antiretroviral treatment. Programs need to invest more attention to each step of this cascade, which is equally valid for other chronic diseases and was originally described for tuberculosis control in the 1960s by Maurice Piot.[14] Problems of cost, transport, access to and quality of services, the position of women, and supply of medicines are frequent in some countries, and the situation can be volatile. For example, in 2010 38 percent of low-income countries claimed at least once to be out of stock of antiretrovirals in health centers. Even with free antiretrovirals for patients, adherence may not be guaranteed. Some countries such as Uganda, Botswana, Kenya, and South Africa, and organizations such as MSF and TASO, proposed ways to improve adherence and follow-up. They notably consist of bringing delivery points closer to patients, associating family members or neighbors with patient support, elite adherence clubs, contracts between patient and health personnel, and incentives such as adherence vouchers for transport costs. Last but not least, stigma associated with HIV continues to be one of the major obstacles to treatment access, uptake, and adherence, besides being an endemic violation of human rights.

With significant prolongation of life thanks to antiretroviral treatment, people living with HIV often experience accelerated ageing processes. Co-morbidity with pathology of metabolism and bone density, and in the cardiovascular, hepatic, and renal systems, is increasingly complicating care, and will be particularly difficult to address in poor resource environments. Simplified and affordable strategies should be urgently developed for these new clinical challenges.

Health services of countries with a high burden of HIV are struggling with an ever-rising number of people on chronic antiretroviral treatment. New and more efficient health care delivery modes will be necessary to cope with chronic care for millions, not only for AIDS, but also for the growing number of patients with other chronic diseases.

Health services of countries with a high burden of HIV are struggling with an ever-rising number of people on chronic antiretroviral treatment. New and more efficient health care delivery modes will be necessary to cope with chronic care for millions, not only for AIDS, but also for the growing number of patients with other chronic diseases.[15] There is an urgent need to redesign HIV care delivery through new approaches. These include standardization and simplification of treatment regimens and procedures, decentralization and integration into mainstream health services, and "task shifting" (with less skilled health workers performing tasks currently delivered by scarcer and more expensive clinicians). That such task shifting can be effective was shown in a study in Uganda,[16] where local TASO volunteers were as effective as doctors and nurses for follow-up, and at much less cost to the patient. Another study in Uganda showed that the rates of virological failure in patients followed in health centers or at home were comparable.[17] Furthermore, in a multicenter study in Africa mortality under treatment was no greater with a simplified approach to CD4 cell monitoring than with routine laboratory testing.[18] Nevertheless more research is needed to determine whether monitoring viral load with simplified techniques will be necessary for long-term antiretroviral treatment, given the inevitable development of antiretroviral resistance. Another challenge is to offer dual therapy for HIV and tuberculosis, a very frequent co-infection, although only about half of tuberculosis patients worldwide were tested for HIV.

In the long term the cost of second- and third-line treatment and the proportion of patients needing it because of the development of antiretroviral resistance are unknown. Second- and third-line drugs are used when patients develop a "failure of therapy," where the first-line regimen is not effective anymore. This can happen if, for example, the first-line drugs were not taken correctly, allowing the virus to develop resistance them. Such second- and third-line drugs are typically more expensive, and generic versions are often not available. Standardized treatment regimens and support for adherence are the best ways to prevent resistance, but the development of new drugs is vital given the high mutation rate of HIV and frequent operational and behavioral challenges. Today between 2 and 10 percent of those receiving antiretroviral therapy are on second-line drugs. For example, in Brazil the national cost of treatment doubled in five years because of increased need for second-line medication. The annual cost of first-line antiretroviral drugs was about one hundred fifty dollars to two hundred dollars, as compared to fifteen hundred dollars or more for second-line drugs in sub-Saharan Africa.

Whereas spectacular progress has been achieved globally in terms of access to antiretroviral treatment for adults, there are still important research and practical questions that require immediate and long-term attention. Optimization of treatment in terms of type of drugs, dosage, and costs remains necessary. One key area is access to pediatric antiretroviral treatment, which is still inadequate and the medication badly adapted to infants and children. Simple and inexpensive point of care diagnostics for HIV viral load are also needed. On the funding side, long-term dependence on international aid for the survival of sometimes hundreds of thousands of citizens under antiretroviral treatment is a high risk for many African states. It even puts into question sovereignty when the survival of so many depends on a vote in the U.S. Congress or a decision by another donor country.

> As Ethan Kapstein wrote, the AIDS movement transformed antiretrovirals "from private goods into merit goods." A key question is whether greater access to patented drugs for HIV infection has led to access to new medicines to treat other diseases in low- and middle-income countries.

As Ethan Kapstein wrote, the AIDS movement transformed antiretrovirals "from private goods into merit goods."[19] A key question is whether greater access to patented drugs for HIV infection has led to access to new medicines to treat other diseases in low- and middle-income countries. The jury is still out. The next obstacle to access to medicines may be bilateral trade agreements between the United States and individual countries that are much more restrictive in terms of the use of generic pharmaceuticals than what was agreed at the WTO.

Finding a true cure, that is eliminating HIV from the body or fully controlling the virus after stopping therapy, would be a true game changer. However, except for a few individuals in whom this was achieved through either stem cell transplant or very early treatment with complex drug cocktails, the prospect of an affordable cure for large-scale use does not seem to be realistic in the near future. Finally, it is unlikely that we will "treat ourselves out of this epidemic," and intensifying HIV combination prevention will be as crucial as antiretroviral treatment to ultimately bring the epidemic under control.

6

COMBINATION PREVENTION

The search for simple solutions to stop the exponential spread of the HIV epidemic, as with the search for a vaccine, began early. However, a better understanding of the biology, transmission dynamics, and behavioral and structural determinants, combined with results of community and clinical trials, strongly suggest that only a *combination* of behavioral, biological, structural, and antiretroviral approaches can further reduce new HIV infections to low endemic levels—that is until an effective and affordable vaccine becomes widely available.[1] Just as for other public health activities, HIV prevention must be based as far as possible on scientific evidence. However, in practice progress in the fight against AIDS has been the result of synergy among scientific discovery, political engagement, and services on the ground. In the end, politics often made the difference.

Current practices in HIV prevention are the result of thirty years of experience and scientific advances. The first successes were obtained thanks to social mobilization of gay communities in Western countries, as well as in Uganda and Thailand in the early 1990s. Since 1986 national programs for needle and syringe exchange in The Netherlands, the United Kingdom, and Australia have demonstrated their efficacy in reducing HIV transmission among injecting drug users. Prevention of transmission from mother to child using antiretrovirals has been shown since 1998. After years of debate, in 2005 a first trial of male circumcision at Orange Farm in South Africa confirmed a reduction of over 50 percent in the acquisition of HIV from women to circumcised men.

Globally, the number of new HIV infections started to decline near the end of the 1990s, well before the widespread availability of antiretrovirals. However, in 2013 there were still as many as 2.1 million new infections, including 1.5 million in sub-Saharan Africa.

Another milestone was the demonstration in 2010 in South Africa that a microbicide gel with tenofovir reduced the risk of HIV infection in women by 39 percent (54 percent with high gel adherence).[2] Numerous earlier trials with other products had revealed an absence of protection or, worse, increased HIV acquisition in women. Finally, oral pre-exposure prophylaxis (PrEP) was shown to reduce the risk of HIV infection in several populations across the world (though not in every study) with up to 90 percent protection in those who consistently used PrEP.[3]

Globally, the number of new HIV infections started to decline near the end of the 1990s, well before the widespread availability of antiretrovirals. However, in 2012 there were still as many as 2.3 million new infections, including 1.6 million in sub-Saharan Africa. In addition, progress has been very uneven in different countries and populations, and *average* national progress can mask major differences *within* countries, which should not come as a surprise since the HIV pandemic is made up of numerous smaller epidemics, each requiring specific approaches for prevention. Furthermore, worldwide there are still more new infections annually than people with new access to antiretroviral therapy. As a result the gap between those who receive treatment and those in need widens with time.

As we saw in chapter 1, transmission dynamics of infectious diseases can be explained in a simple formula:[4] $R^\circ = \beta c D$. R° is the reproductive rate of an epidemic. This reproductive rate is the result of a combination of β (the probability of transmission), c (the frequency of exposure), and D (the duration of infectivity). If R° exceeds 1 the number of new infections will continue to increase (in other words generate an epidemic); if it is around 1 the infection is endemic; and below 1 the epidemic will decline. This model also indicates the options to interrupt transmission, in other words what kind of interventions can prevent HIV. For example, condom use, male circumcision, avoidance of high-risk practices such as anal sex, needle exchange programs, and antiretroviral medication all influence the probability of transmission from an infected to an uninfected person. A reduction in the number of partners, and in sexual violence, alcohol and drug abuse, and an increase in faithfulness reduce c; antiretroviral therapy and behavioral interventions to increase treatment adherence reduce D. When applying this formula, it is important to recognize that the risk for HIV transmission is not evenly distributed in a population, and that the effectiveness of prevention may vary with risk situation.

GLOBAL, BUT NOT UNIVERSAL, DECLINES IN HIV INCIDENCE

In the 1980s in response to a devastating HIV epidemic in the homosexual communities of Western countries, a significant fall in new infections was obtained at a time when treatment did not exist. This was the result of changes in sexual behavior including a reduction in the number of partners and increased condom use. Thanks to their innovative "100 percent condom" campaign and strong leadership, Thailand was successful in reducing HIV incidence among its heterosexual population, though continuing high infection rates persist among men who have sex with men, as well as among injecting drug users. Uganda was the first African country to experience a decline in new HIV infections as a result of strong leadership and community action around abstinence, faithfulness, and condom use.

Between 2001 and 2011 new infections dropped more than 50 percent in twenty-five countries, including thirteen sub-Saharan African countries, and another nine experienced a decline of at least one third.[5] The worst epidemics, such as in Nigeria, Ethiopia, South Africa, Zambia, and Zimbabwe, were stabilized or showed signs of decline. Reductions in HIV incidence were particularly striking in young people. Thus in Kenya, between 2000 and 2005 there was a 60 percent decline in prevalence among the young, and in South Africa among women aged between fifteen and twenty-four HIV incidence dropped from 5.5 percent between 2003 and 2005 to 2.2 percent in 2005 to 2008—though still an extraordinarily high figure. Many studies, though not all, also document a reduction in high-risk behavior among young people.

In India, thanks to efforts by the National AIDS Control Organisation (NACO), the Avahan project supported by the Gates Foundation, and numerous NGOs, HIV preventive services reach more than 80 percent of sex workers in the most affected states. Between 2003 and 2006 HIV prevalence among Indian sex workers fell by half, from 10 to 5 percent. In Southern India the infection rate in fifteen- to twenty-four-year-old pregnant women dropped from 2 percent to less than 1 percent between 2000 and 2010.

Not all regions followed this trend. A major exception is Eastern Europe, in particular the former Soviet republics, where HIV incidence grew more than 25 percent between 2001 and 2012. In North America and Western Europe, as well as increasingly in Asia and Africa, new infections among men who have sex with men are either stable or increasing. For example, in England the number of new infections doubled in ten years, mainly in homosexual men, with five new infections in gay men every day in London alone in 2013.

MEASURING THE IMPACT OF HIV PREVENTION

A question is raised regularly as to whether the decline in new HIV infections and in prevalence is the result of efforts at prevention and change in sexual behavior, or if it corresponds to the natural history of HIV because those most at risk are already infected or dead. In this context an important observation is that transmission patterns are still evolving, even if there has not been a fundamental change in those who are at highest risk for infection—men who have sex with men and injecting drug users across the world, and sex workers and mobile populations in some countries. For example, Cambodia saw a vast heterosexual

A question is raised regularly as to whether the decline in new HIV infections and in prevalence is the result of efforts at prevention and change in sexual behavior, or if it corresponds to the natural history of HIV because those most at risk are already infected or dead. In this context an important observation is that transmission patterns are still evolving, even if there has not been a fundamental change in those who are at highest risk for infection—men who have sex with men and injecting drug users across the world, and sex workers and mobile populations in some countries.

epidemic in the 1990s, but thanks to intensive condom promotion programs, in a few years the drop in new infections was spectacular. At the start of the epidemic most infections were among sex workers and their clients, then it was the wives and noncommercial partners of infected men, and finally the children of infected women. Similarly, in several Eastern and Central African countries most new transmissions are now within stable couples, during casual sex, and among men who have sex with men, while transmission during commercial sex continues, though proportionally less than before. In Ukraine the epidemic continues to be dominated by transmission through injecting drug use, mainly in men. However, the percentage of women with HIV has increased consistently due to transmission by drug users to their female sex partners. Thus in 2009, 45 percent of people living with HIV in Ukraine were women compared with 37 percent in 1999 and less than 20 percent at the beginning of the epidemic.[6]

A further complication is that there is no reliable biological test to measure HIV incidence (new infections in a given time) on a large scale, and long-term data on new infections in a population to estimate progress of the epidemic are rarely available. Incidence is more difficult to determine than prevalence, in the first place because it is a much smaller figure, meaning that large sample sizes are needed, and errors in measurement may be higher than when estimating prevalence. Estimating incidence is essential to understand recent transmission dynamics of HIV, as this is where efforts for prevention should be directed in order to have an impact on future infections. Prevalence and incidence may not always evolve in the same direction. For example, paradoxically, prevalence has increased in countries where generalized access to antiretroviral therapy allows people with HIV to live longer, even when the incidence remains stable. The gold standard in measuring HIV incidence is to follow a cohort of uninfected individuals over a long period. Regular testing then reveals new infections. These longitudinal studies are long, laborious, and costly, and usually do not respond to the immediate needs of HIV prevention programs.

Complex mathematical models are useful to estimate incidence from prevalence, as done by UNAIDS, and to test hypotheses about the impact of several factors on observed fluctuations in prevalence. For example, Tim Hallett and colleagues[7] at Imperial College London showed that a decline in HIV prevalence in a number of African countries cannot be explained only by the natural history of the epidemic, but also implies changes in sexual behavior.

Another example is the evolution of HIV in Zimbabwe, in political turmoil for several decades. Prevalence was an astonishing 24 percent in adults at the end of the 1990s and the incidence had reached 6 percent per year in adults. Since the 2000s acceleration in the decline of new infections was probably due to change in sexual behavior (figure 6.1). Whereas during the political and economic crisis HIV prevention programs continued to be financed externally, a major decline in disposable income, forced immobility, and insecurity may have resulted in a reduction in high-risk behavior, contributing to the fall in incidence.

Demonstrating the impact of prevention programs ideally requires randomized controlled trials, which compare an intervention with a control group. Whereas these are essential to establish the efficacy of new biomedical interventions, they are rarely able to evaluate large-scale programs, and have their limits in assessing the effectiveness of more complex behavioral and structural prevention programs. In such cases, a combination of quantitative and qualitative methods is probably the best option to evaluate the impact of programs.

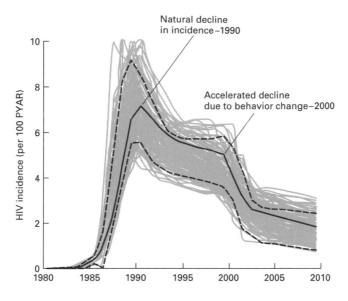

FIGURE 6.1 TRENDS IN NEW HIV INFECTIONS IN ZIMBABWE, 1980–2010.

SOURCE: HALLETT ET AL. 2009.

COMBINATION PREVENTION

A recurrent myth in HIV prevention is that there is a single solution to stopping its spread, such as male circumcision,[8] reduction of the number of concomitant partners,[9] or screening of a whole population followed by antiretroviral therapy of all individuals found to be infected.[10] Not recognizing the complexity of AIDS not only reflects a lack of

> If we have learned one lesson over the last thirty years it is that there is no silver bullet for HIV prevention. Only a combination of interventions, adapted to the local level, with sufficient coverage, adherence, and duration, have an optimal impact on the spread of HIV—in other words "combination prevention."

scientific rigor, it can even be dangerous as it diverts limited resources to ineffective approaches. If we have learned one lesson over the last thirty years it is that there is no silver bullet for HIV prevention. Only a combination of interventions, adapted to the local level, with sufficient coverage, adherence, and duration, have an optimal impact on the spread of HIV—in other words "combination prevention."[11]

Combination prevention requires simultaneous action on several fronts. This includes condom use, behavioral change toward fidelity and fewer sex partners, smaller age differences between partners, male circumcision in high-prevalence countries, antiretroviral therapy including PrEP, harm reduction through substitution therapy and access to clean needles and syringes for injecting drug users, structural interventions against sexual violence and alcohol abuse, and countering HIV-related stigma. Each specific epidemiological situation should be addressed through an optimal combination of interventions. The concept of combination prevention is not new in public health or social programs,[12] though it has been less popular in infectious disease control. For example, anti-smoking and obesity campaigns are using it. A key question for HIV prevention is the effectiveness of various combinations for a given risk situation, and more research is needed in this area.

FOCUS ON HIGH-RISK SITUATIONS

In addition to using a combination of interventions, a focus on high HIV transmission areas and populations should be a priority as such an approach is likely to generate the most impact on a very heterogeneous epidemic. In addition, it is important to recognize considerable overlap between high-risk groups and geography. For example, whereas in Kenya approximately 40 percent of new infections occur in HIV-discordant couples, in the capital Nairobi and on the coast, men who have sex with men contribute to a growing proportion of new infections. So the epidemic is still evolving and, from a historic perspective, possibly still in a relatively early phase in a number of countries. Thus whereas in Africa heterosexual transmission clearly dominates, HIV spread among men who have sex with men is becoming better documented, and in countries such as Kenya, Tanzania, Zanzibar, Nigeria, Senegal, and South Africa transmission associated with injecting drug use is emerging.

Resources are often not used where transmission is happening because of reluctance to invest in programs for stigmatized and marginalized populations. For example, in Eastern Europe and Central Asia UNAIDS estimated that about 90 percent of AIDS funding did not address the most affected groups, such as drug users, men who have sex with men, and sex workers and their clients. Similarly in Kenya and Mozambique, where 25 to 30 percent of new infections are in these populations, less than 0.5 percent of the AIDS budget goes to them. Likewise in Asia funding of prevention in these populations is less than 10 percent, with a few exceptions like Cambodia. In Latin America, except in Peru, Brazil, and Argentina, there is a major gap between prevention funding and the needs of communities of homosexual men, where prevalence is 20 to 30 percent. In Costa Rica homosexual men represent 60 percent of HIV cases, whereas their budget for prevention is less than 1 percent of the total AIDS budget. In Panama the figures are about 40 percent and 2 percent, and in Guatemala 35 percent and 4 percent, respectively.[13] It should not come as a surprise that HIV prevention is not working in these populations! It is also the case in the large towns of Asia such as in China (5 percent of people with HIV), Indonesia (9 percent), Vietnam (4 percent), and Laos (5 percent). In Africa, where homosexuality remains a great taboo, very high rates of infection among gay men have been revealed in the large towns of South Africa (15 percent), Kenya (13 percent), Malawi (21 percent), and Dakar (22 percent). Many homosexual men in Africa and Asia are married and when infected may infect their wives, with whom they rarely use a condom. In Central Asia, Africa, and the Caribbean, where homophobia is strongly embedded, major structural and cultural changes are needed, such as decriminalization of homosexuals and establishment of services for them.[14]

Even where HIV prevention was successful, trends may reverse. This is currently happening in Europe and the United States, which are experiencing either an increased number of new infections in homosexual men, or the lack of a significant decrease (figure 6.2). In the United

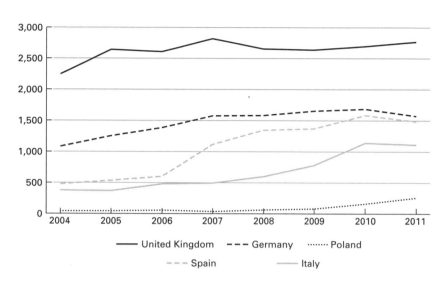

FIGURE 6.2 NUMBER OF NEW HIV DIAGNOSES AMONG MEN WHO HAVE SEX WITH
MEN IN THE UK, GERMANY, POLAND, SPAIN, AND ITALY, 2004–2011.

Source: HIV/AIDS surveillance in Europe 2011, European Centre for Disease Prevention and Control
(ECDC), and the World Health Organization Regional Office for Europe 2012, ECDC, Stockholm.

States the situation is particularly dramatic among African American
homosexual men. We must urgently match HIV prevention better to
people and places. The "cookie cutter approach" should be abandoned
for more locally driven programs—obviously guided by scientific evidence on the various components and their combination to prevent
HIV infection.

ANTIRETROVIRAL TREATMENT AS PREVENTION

A landmark trial published in 2011 demonstrated that early antiretroviral
treatment of the infected partner in stable discordant couples reduced
HIV transmission by as much as 96 percent, as compared to deferring
treatment until clinically indicated.[15] There was also clinical benefit of
early initiation of antiretroviral therapy, since this resulted in about a

40 percent lower rate of adverse reactions. It has been known for a while that viral load in plasma and genital secretions is the major determinant predicting sexual transmission of HIV.[16] Treatment as prevention is based on a reduction of infectiousness by a reduction of blood and genital concentrations of virus through antiretroviral medication, and the same principle has been applied for two decades to prevent HIV transmission from mother to child. All this means that there is an additional benefit of antiretroviral treatment beyond its primary aim to improve the health of people living with HIV. Interestingly, a similar study[17] among HIV-discordant couples in Uganda did not find any difference, though antiretroviral therapy was provided only to the infected partners when their CD4+ lymphocyte levels were below two hundred fifty per mm3 (indicating more advanced immunodeficiency), and it is unclear how comparable the two studies are.

A key question now is whether treatment as prevention can reduce HIV transmission at the population level, in other words, whether clinical efficacy is translated into real-world effectiveness. Whereas an ecological study in KwaZulu-Natal Province in South Africa found a 34 percent decline in HIV incidence in populations with 30 to 40 percent coverage by antiretroviral treatment as compared to areas with less than 10 percent coverage, in neighboring Swaziland incidence continues at a very high level of 2.4 percent per year despite one of the highest antiretroviral treatment rates in sub-Saharan Africa of 85 percent. At the same time HIV incidence continues unchanged or is rising in highly treated communities of men who have sex with men in Western countries, suggesting at least that the impact for prevention of antiretroviral treatment in these communities is either very limited or nonexistent. Controlled community trials in Africa, North America, and Europe are currently assessing the effectiveness of early treatment for population-level HIV prevention.

If antiretroviral treatment is adopted for large-scale HIV prevention, a number of complex operational questions will have to be addressed, as well as the challenge of a significant boost in funding when resources for HIV activities are stagnating. Acceptability of chronic treatment in healthy people living with HIV (for example, in one study 30 percent of discordant couples deferred early antiretroviral treatment when offered), as well as crucial treatment adherence and the risk of development of resistance are particularly challenging. Finally, the ethics of offering preventive antiretroviral treatment can be questioned when a majority of people living with HIV who are eligible for treatment on clinical and immunological grounds have still no access.

PRE-EXPOSURE PROPHYLAXIS AS PREVENTION

Pre-exposure prophylaxis (PrEP) for HIV prevention is the use of antiretroviral medication before sex. It is based on the same principles as anti-malaria prophylaxis or antibiotic therapy before surgery, and the prevention of mother-to-child transmission is also partly based on it, since the fetus or infant is given medication before or during exposure to HIV from the mother.

A trial in South Africa was the first to demonstrate that a vaginal gel with 1 percent tenofovir reduced acquisition of HIV on average by nearly 40 percent in women, and even more when used consistently.[18] Subsequent trials showed that oral prophylaxis with tenofovir, with or without emtricitabine, protected homosexual men, and heterosexual women and men by 44 to 73 percent. However, two clinical trials did not find such protection.[19] Not surprisingly, efficacy of PrEP depends on adherence to the medication: in other words, PrEP works when used.

In 2013 the U.S. Food and Drug Administration approved daily use of oral tenofovir and emtricitabine for PrEP to prevent sexually acquired HIV infection in adults at high risk. Before PrEP can be recommended for global use, some important issues for policy and implementation should be addressed, such as the cost effectiveness in specific populations, promotion and sustaining of adherence to prophylactic medication, and possibly the risk of development of resistance. In general, it seems that PrEP should become part of combination prevention in populations at highest risk for HIV, but more user-friendly regimens such as intercourse-related PrEP would probably increase its real world impact.

MALE CIRCUMCISION AS PREVENTION

Male circumcision is a lifelong and fairly effective intervention to prevent HIV acquisition in men through vaginal intercourse, with a protection of approximately 50 percent.[20] This trial, performed in South Africa in 2005 by Auvert and colleagues, and confirmed by others in Kenya and Uganda, ended a fifteen-year controversy as to the importance of male circumcision as a biological determinant for HIV spread, at least partially explaining differences in prevalence between various African populations. The first epidemiological study[21] suggesting a protective effect of male circumcision was made in Nairobi in the 1980s, followed by dozens of other studies in Africa, most of which showed an association between HIV risk and lack of male circumcision. On the other hand the low rate of male circumcision in Europe did not provoke a large epidemic. As male circumcision is in the first place linked to culture, tradition, and religion, which may all act as major confounders for HIV acquisition, it was not possible to conclude unequivocally that it protects against infection unless controlled clinical trials were performed. Unfortunately it took over a decade before such trials were funded. An additional benefit of male circumcision is that it also lowers the incidence of genital ulcers and infection with human papillomavirus, a cause of cervical and head and neck cancers. However, male circumcision does not lower HIV risk for women during intercourse.

As a result of this conclusive research African countries with a severe HIV epidemic have launched massive circumcision programs. Except for Nyanza Province in Kenya, where now over 60 percent of eligible men have been circumcised, mass circumcision programs are lagging far behind their targets in nearly all countries. Recent development of devices to perform male circumcision without surgery and stronger support among traditional and political leaders may change this implementation challenge. It is still not clear whether circumcised men will use condoms less frequently in the belief that they are protected, as a decline in condom use could wipe out the benefits of circumcision. Neonatal circumcision seems to be the best option in the long term, as it is less cumbersome and expensive, and will protect as of the first intercourse in life. In the meantime, male circumcision should be an integral part of combination prevention in populations where this is traditionally not practiced and the risk of HIV is high.

PREVENTION OF MOTHER-TO-CHILD TRANSMISSION OF HIV

In 1994 the Pediatric AIDS Clinical Trials Group 076 Study demonstrated for the first time that the transmission of HIV from mother to child can be prevented. The trial showed that zidovudine (AZT) can reduce mother-to-child transmission by 67 percent in the absence of breastfeeding.[22] In the meantime more effective regimens for prophylaxis of mother-to-child transmission have been developed, and the current WHO recommendation is to offer pregnant women living with HIV standard first-line therapy with tenofovir, 3TC, and efavirenz, and then stop one week after complete cessation of breastfeeding if there is no clinical indication to continue antiretroviral treatment for the mother, while also giving nevirapine to the breastfed infant.[23]

Prevention of mother-to-child transmission of HIV was initially judged inapplicable in low-income countries, where the need was greatest. Highly recommended breastfeeding practically reversed the advantages of perinatal antiretroviral therapy in mother and child as breast milk may also contain high concentrations of HIV. In poor populations facing infectious diseases and inferior health services, breastfeeding until twelve months was best for infant survival, even if born with HIV. In high-income countries the use of infant formula, quality obstetric care, prophylactic cesarean section, general access to antiretroviral treatment, and ever-improved prophylactic antiretrovirals have reduced the risk of mother-to-child transmission in less than 1.5 percent of cases since the beginning of the 2000s. It is not the same in much of sub-Saharan Africa where mother-to-child transmission remains around 20 percent in several countries. Although lack of access to antenatal services offering diagnosis and treatment, and stigma associated with HIV are the two main obstacles to the elimination of mother-to-child transmission, the dilemma of breastfeeding is a major additional obstacle when full anti-retroviral coverage of the lactating mother and infant are not available.

In 2013, 54 percent of pregnant women in low- and middle-income countries did not receive an HIV test. Sixty-eight percent of pregnant women living with HIV received antiretroviral prophylaxis in 2013, compared to 15 percent in 2005: real progress. Some countries, like Botswana, South Africa, Namibia and Swaziland reach more than 90 percent coverage, while others like Nigeria Chad and the Democratic Republic of the Congo are closer to 30 percent coverage or lower.[24] The main reasons for poor performance are related to the low availability of antenatal consultation. In the twenty countries with the greatest number of HIV-positive pregnant women the percentage of those tested and counseled ranges from over 90 percent in South Africa and Zambia to 9 percent in the Democratic Republic of the Congo. UN agencies and the U.S. government have been calling for elimination of HIV infection in neonates, for an "AIDS-free generation," which is theoretically possible in many settings, but the practical obstacles are enormous, particularly in some African countries.

HIV PREVENTION IN INJECTING DRUG USERS

Harm reduction programs for injecting drug users can be highly effective to prevent HIV transmission. Harm reduction aims to minimize the adverse health, social, and economic consequences of drug use, without necessarily eliminating drug consumption. They basically combine substitution therapy for opiate addiction with a longer-acting and less euphoric opioid (usually methadone or buprenorphine, and in a few countries heroin maintenance provided by the state), availability of clean syringes and needles, and access to HIV and addiction treatment. The success of anti-drug policies is measured by reduction in the number of drug users; the success of harm reduction programs is measured by decrease in deaths, disease, HIV and hepatitis B and C infections, and drug-related crime.

Harm reduction has often clashed with classic anti-drug policies aimed at stopping drug use, with zero tolerance for consumption of illicit drugs. The concept of harm reduction appeared in Great Britain, The Netherlands, and Australia in the mid-1980s. It is part of a tradition of public health policies based on a certain pragmatic acceptance of drug use and risk-taking behavior. It can be summarized in the following cascade: Best not to consume drugs, but if you do, better consume the least dangerous ones; best not to inject drugs, but if you do, use a sterile syringe. Since 1990 Switzerland has adopted this new approach, with anti-addiction policies based on four pillars: prevention of drug use, treatment of addiction, harm reduction, and law enforcement. Harm reduction has been shown in numerous studies to decrease the incidence of new HIV infections among injecting drug users, though its effectiveness may be negatively affected in populations injecting cocaine and synthetic drugs, often in combination.[25] Importantly, trials showed that needle exchange did not cause an increase in injecting drug use.

Outside sub-Saharan Africa, HIV transmission through injecting drugs represents one third of new cases of HIV infection. In Eastern Europe and Central Asia, where the HIV epidemic is still expanding, it is by far the leading factor. Studies have also shown that purely repressive measures may actually contribute to the spread of HIV, since drug users stay underground as much as possible, continue to share needles and syringes, have unprotected sex, and often avoid social services. Ukraine is one of the rare former Soviet states to have applied large-scale harm reduction, though with regular variations in policy and implementation. As a result it has managed to stabilize HIV prevalence at 1.1 percent—still the highest in Europe. Since then the proportion of Ukrainians contracting the virus sexually exceeds that infected by injection: 43 percent versus 35 percent in 2009.

Yet only 15 percent of countries confronted with an HIV epidemic among drug users have adopted effective policies. The refusal of many governments (such as Russia and Thailand) to provide sterile syringes and needles and/or substitution therapy continues to nurture epidemics among drug users. In Russia and several former Soviet states injecting drug users are treated inhumanely: methadone is illegal in many places and government priority is to arrest drug users and place them in prison or detoxification centers with no access to medical care for their addiction. In addition, drug users are severely discriminated against in terms of access to antiretroviral treatment.[26] That policy change in this very politically sensitive domain is possible was dramatically illustrated by the Chinese government in June 2005, when it decided to organize harm reduction programs, in particular through the establishment of hundreds of methadone clinics. However, repressive policies and detoxification centers continue to coexist with harm reduction. In the United States federal policy for support of needle exchange programs has been highly controversial. Federal funding for such programs was banned in 1988, briefly overturned in 2009, but reinstated by Congress in 2011. Of the two hundred needle exchange programs in the United States, about 80 percent are funded by local and state governments. Thanks to a long-standing and early needle exchange program, New York City succeeded in reducing the annual number of HIV infections among drug users from thirteen thousand to about one hundred fifty per year.

Harm reduction is a sad example of a scientifically proven HIV prevention policy hijacked by harmful politics. Above all, it requires political courage more than anything else.

THE POLITICS OF HIV PREVENTION

In spite of scientific advances and a growing number of HIV prevention options, HIV continues to spread throughout the world at a pace of well over two million new cases per year. Major reasons for very slow progress in HIV prevention have been lack of political will, insufficient funds, and poor technical and strategic leadership.

In general,[27] whenever we made good progress in the struggle against AIDS it has been largely thanks to good political decisions. On the contrary, bad or no decisions have consistently led to more HIV infections and deaths. Governments delays in providing access to antiretrovirals because of denialist beliefs, such as in South Africa under President Mbeki, reluctance by international donors to invest in HIV prevention and treatment, opposition to condom use or harm reduction for drug users, and laws to prohibit homosexuality, are all examples of damaging

> In general, HIV prevention is far more controversial than access to antiretroviral therapy, because of its association with moral and religious beliefs and societal traditions. As such it requires extraordinary leadership in each society to ensure that lives are protected using the best available scientific evidence and considerations of social justice, while sometimes going against mainstream public opinion. Such leadership may mean the difference between life and death for many citizens, particularly the more vulnerable ones.

decisions for HIV prevention and treatment. They reflect the uneasiness of political, religious, and other leaders, and large fractions of society, when faced with an epidemic driven by sex and drugs. In general, HIV prevention is far more controversial than access to antiretroviral therapy, because of its association with moral and religious beliefs and societal traditions. As such it requires extraordinary leadership in each society to ensure that lives are protected using the best available scientific evidence and considerations of social justice, while sometimes going against mainstream public opinion. Such leadership may mean the difference between life and death for many citizens, particularly the more vulnerable ones.

In addition there are daily operational challenges to implement even the most straightforward interventions when basic services are inadequate. Thus even a relatively simple and low-cost intervention such as prevention of mother-to-child transmission has been very slow to reach a majority of women and infants in need. As mentioned earlier, misallocation of limited resources for HIV prevention as a result of negative politics or poor technical leadership may also result in ineffective programs. HIV prevention is yet another illustration that scientific evidence does not automatically lead to action. For example, the Framework Convention on Tobacco Control (FCTC) was adopted by the WHO in 2003, more than fifty years after Richard Doll and Austin Bradford Hill proved the link between tobacco and lung cancer.[28]

STRUCTURAL DETERMINANTS AND SEXUAL VIOLENCE

There are a number of behaviors and structural determinants that can indirectly have a major impact on the course of HIV epidemics and the response to them.[29] Vulnerability to HIV infection is multifactorial: it is influenced by gender inequality, unemployment, poverty, access to social support, education level, and human rights. HIV-related stigmatization and discrimination also contribute to increasing vulnerability, including by blocking access to prevention, testing, and treatment. AIDS programs must take this complexity into account by adapting priorities to each situation: legal reform might be the determining factor in one situation while in another stopping police violence against drug users could be critical.

Violence against women is widespread and has been identified consistently as increasing the risk of HIV infection.[30] For example, in the Eastern Cape province of South Africa a study[31] showed that young female victims of sexual violence by their partner had little power over their sex life and HIV protection, and were more susceptible to HIV infection than other women. Similarly, homophobic violence is endemic in many societies and is a major obstacle to HIV programs for homosexual men.

Structural approaches to HIV prevention are an essential part of combination prevention, though their exact nature and prioritization depend on the local context. Examples are programs to reduce violence against women and cash transfers.[32] In the latter case cash payments can be used for food, education, health care, and transport, and a controlled study in Malawi showed that giving cash of the equivalent of ten dollars per month to adolescents girls if they worked well at school led to a fall of 40 percent in early marriage, 30 percent in unwanted pregnancies, and 38 percent in early sexual activity, compared to a control group. Another measure was to provide education and microfinancing to poor women in rural South Africa.[33] Two years later violence by the male partner had fallen by 55 percent, but there was no effect on condom use or HIV incidence. As alcohol abuse is related to both sex-based violence and risk of HIV, it is important to evaluate interventions as to their impact on risk, and include such approaches into combination prevention.

Changing social norms relevant to HIV prevention may take years. Besides their cultural and political sensitivity, the long lead time may be a major reason they are usually neglected. There is a need to invest more in these programs and to be ready to persevere for a decade if necessary to see any results. Priorities in this domain are gender-based violence and the end of legal and social discrimination of homosexuality.

Another example in Kenya[34] illustrates the importance of structural factors. In an environment in which 15 percent of eighteen-year-old girls were infected with HIV, eight times more than boys of the same age, providing free school uniforms to school girls resulted in better school results and fewer pregnancies, compared to girls who had to pay for their uniform, as was the norm. Another effective intervention was to inform school girls about the relative risks of sex with older men compared to sex with boys of their age. This resulted in fewer unwanted pregnancies.

Changing social norms relevant to HIV prevention may take years. Besides their cultural and political sensitivity, the long lead time may be a major reason they are usually neglected. There is a need to invest more in these programs and to be ready to persevere for a decade if necessary to see any results. Priorities in this domain are gender-based violence and the end of legal and social discrimination of homosexuality.[35] The aids2031 Consortium proposed a minimum legal framework for all countries including decriminalization of HIV infection and transmission, prostitution, and same-sex relations. This framework should also remove barriers that prevent harm reduction services for injecting drug users.

Finally, a supportive legal environment is essential for the success of any HIV program.[36] Laws that ban harm reduction for injecting drug users, prohibit same-sex relations, drive prostitution underground, or limit condom promotion are all major obstacles for HIV prevention. Even where a supportive legal environment exists, there may still be a lack of enforcement of the law, undermining AIDS programs.

There may be a short window of opportunity to greatly intensify combination prevention and antiretroviral treatment before control of the pandemic evolves beyond our fiscal and interventional means. Beside resolute local and international leadership, this renewed effort in HIV prevention will also require a strategic and operational renaissance.

A RENAISSANCE IN HIV PREVENTION

Poor commitment and leadership remain the biggest obstacles to effective large-scale HIV prevention across the world. In recent years efforts concentrated on access to treatment, which was essential to save millions of people living with HIV. The finding that antiretroviral treatment also reduces the risk of transmission has led to claims that the end of the epidemic is near. Whereas the end of AIDS and the HIV epidemic should clearly be our collective aspiration, it is unlikely that this will happen with current tools and level of effort, in particular as long as an effective vaccine is not available. What is achievable in the next decade or so is converting the HIV pandemic into low endemic levels of infection in most societies and communities. At the same time research and innovation need to continue to improve HIV prevention, including the development of a preventive vaccine.[37]

Recent experience has shown that progress in HIV prevention can be fragile and reversible, as seen in countries such as Uganda and in communities of men who have sex with men in North America and Europe. Therefore there may be a short window of opportunity to greatly intensify combination prevention and antiretroviral treatment before control of the pandemic evolves beyond our fiscal and interventional means. Beside resolute local and international leadership, this renewed effort in HIV prevention will also require a strategic and operational renaissance. We must recognize the limitations of individual interventions and tools, apply the most effective combination of interventions for each micro-epidemic, focus resources on the geography of high transmission and vulnerable populations, drastically improve program delivery, and regularly adapt strategies and interventions when epidemic drivers evolve.[38] A strategic change in this direction should obviously capitalize on current achievements, but will require some fundamental restructuring of effort.

7

THE ECONOMICS OF AIDS

A
s for any health issue, HIV infection has major economic dimensions. In addition to its social and public health aspects, the economic impact of AIDS, as well as the costs of controlling it, are important arguments to put it on national and international political agendas.

ECONOMIC DRIVERS OF THE AIDS EPIDEMIC

In general the poor are more affected by disease than the rich. It is the case for infant mortality, cardiovascular disease, diabetes, tuberculosis, and maternal mortality across the world. As is often the case, AIDS is different. The association between economic status and the disease seems more complex, probably because sex is the main route of transmission, transgressing classic disease vulnerabilities that are largely determined by social context and access to health services. Whereas the poorest region in the world is sub-Saharan Africa, which is also the region most affected by HIV, the richest subregion, Southern Africa, has the highest HIV infection rate. Economic inequality within a society as measured by the Gini coefficient—an indicator in which 0 equals absolute equality and 1 absolute inequality—seems to be a stronger determinant of HIV spread than absolute income. In general, HIV prevalence and incidence do not correlate well with the gross domestic product (GDP) of a country, but the correlation is somewhat stronger, though not absolute, for

Gini coefficient and HIV prevalence.[1] Sub-Saharan African countries with the highest level of economic inequality have the highest HIV infection rates, though they are almost all Southern African countries with major mining industries. This association between inequality and HIV spread has only been found in Africa, where most transmission is heterosexual and where prevalence exceeds 2 percent in the adult population. More equal societies, with better balanced social capital and perhaps more resilience, may be better able to manage a sexually transmitted epidemic. In countries where the epidemic is concentrated in high-risk groups, as in Europe, Asia, and the Americas, the epidemic affects all social classes, though anecdotic reports from countries such as Vietnam and China mention the three Ms—mobile men with money— as being at higher risk of HIV.

As discussed earlier, the organization of labor in Southern Africa, particularly in the mining sector, probably played a significant role in the spread of HIV. High concentrations of young adults doing dangerous work, living in single-sex compounds, and separated from their families and community provide a unique opportunity for the spread of a sexually transmitted virus such as HIV—particularly under apartheid or the postcolonial era, before prevention and treatment programs were introduced.

Data on the impact of educational levels on the spread of HIV are equally mixed. Thus early reports on the relation between prevalence and educational attainment in sub-Saharan Africa often found that better educated people were more infected than less educated ones. It appeared that men with money often have the most sex partners, though for women this was highly variable by country, and prostitution affects the poorest women more. However, with the development of HIV prevention programs and greater openness about it in society, less educated men and women became relatively more infected than more educated people. In Brazil and Nicaragua in the 1980s, for example, most infected men had secondary or higher education and a better economic status, but since the mid-1990s they only represented one third of new HIV cases. This trend may be due to the more educated and well off responding better to prevention as they have easier access to information and services. They also have better access to treatment.

Inequality of the sexes clearly plays a major role in HIV spread. In sub-Saharan Africa women are more infected than men, especially when young, with adolescent girls infected up to six times more often than boys of the same age. Studies suggest that these young women are often not infected by men of their own age but by older men.

Inequality of the sexes clearly plays a major role in HIV spread. In sub-Saharan Africa women are more infected than men, especially when young, with adolescent girls infected up to six times more often than boys of the same age. Studies suggest that these young women are often not infected by men of their own age but by older men. In addition, violence against women and sexual minorities is widespread, and greatly increases women's and homosexual men's vulnerability to infection.

Economic development can affect the spread of HIV in sometimes paradoxical ways. For example, a major economic decline, as experienced in Zimbabwe, was associated with a decline in prevalence. Unemployment, hunger, and insecurity greatly reduced disposable cash and social life, with men having difficulties in maintaining multiple concomitant relationships. In addition, HIV prevention programs continued to be delivered by community-based organizations with support from the international community. In Asian countries such as China, Vietnam, and Malaysia economic growth may play a role in the spread of HIV, at the same time as growth in commercial sex and drug use.

THE IMPACT OF AIDS ON THE ECONOMY

In severely affected societies, AIDS has an economic impact in terms of human and social capital, households, business, health costs, savings, and investments. During the 1990s the economic impact of AIDS in countries with low HIV prevalence was in general overestimated, and underestimated in Southern Africa. The impact of AIDS is less concentrated in countries where HIV is mainly present in high-risk groups: its impact may be negligible in macroeconomic terms, but severe at the level of a community or a town, for example in the gay population. Its impact on families is well documented, as is its sectoral impact. AIDS does not strike everywhere in the same way. For example, those businesses where the labor force is mobile are most affected.

Macroeconomic Impact of AIDS

Numerous studies on the macroeconomic impact of HIV infection have been published, but they have often had a large margin of error as various levels of impact have not been well quantified, in particular the long-term consequences and ripple effects. With more widespread access to antiretroviral therapy, macro-impact estimates of AIDS seem to have been exaggerated in the past. The World Bank published several studies on the economic effects of the epidemic in Southern Africa, including in Botswana, a country with a population of 1.6 million, where approximately 25 percent of the adult population was living with HIV around the turn of the century before antiretroviral therapy became available. Life expectancy had fallen by twenty-five years and economic development slowed by 1.5 percent per year in the previous decade. Similarly, in Namibia the epidemic had reduced GDP growth by 1.1 percent per year, and in South Africa 0.3 to 0.4 percent.[2] These macroeconomic models are essentially based on a single measure of performance: growth of gross national product (GNP). They may actually underestimate the economic impact of AIDS, notably by not taking into account the difficulty of replacing qualified workers in sectors such as industry, education, or health, and the impact of AIDS on the informal economy. Several

> In addition to a general macroeconomic impact, the loss of transmission of knowledge or social capital from one generation to another and its effects on development were significant in heavily affected communities.

elements should be considered, including direct costs (for example treatment, funerals, and reduced savings), and indirect costs (lost productivity and supply of labor). The demographic impact of the death of young adults was considerable before the availability of treatment.

In addition to a general macroeconomic impact, the loss of transmission of knowledge or social capital from one generation to another and its effects on development were significant in heavily affected communities, again before the advent of antiretroviral treatment. In 2004 the International Labour Organization estimated that "Over time, reduced rates of savings lead to diminished investment, slower growth of aggregate output, constraints on employment, and the likelihood of impoverishment."[3] In some studies AIDS in a household increased the risk of children dropping out of school. Deprived of education and confronted with insecurity these children are at higher risk for HIV themselves.

Some of the first detailed studies on the impact of AIDS on the lives of individuals, families, and communities were conducted from 1991 to 1993 in the Kagera region on Lake Victoria in Tanzania.[4] When a young adult died in a poor family their spending for food fell by more than one third and consumption fell by 15 percent. Among the less poor, expenses increased due to the cost of a funeral. In some cultures the funeral often lasts several weeks and involves considerable expense for the extended family. A whole year's income, or even that of several years, is sometimes needed. When such deaths come early in life, and there are several in a year, AIDS may thus affect the whole of an extended family, which can deplete agricultural production. A study by the Food and Agriculture Organization (FAO) in 2002 in Swaziland on small agricultural undertakings noted a 34 percent reduction in cultivated land, 54 percent in maize production, and 29 percent in livestock in those affected by HIV infection. Rural families in Kenya and Rwanda affected by AIDS sometimes abandoned cash crops in favor of less labor intensive subsistence farming.[5]

In 2002 in South Africa health care costs might represent an average of 34 percent of the monthly income of households with a member living with AIDS, whereas the national average was 4 percent. Half the families interviewed reported shortage of food, especially in rural areas.

Some families had to sell their few possessions, livestock, or land, thus impoverishing several generations. In India, for those who had no access to antiretroviral treatment, the financial burden of AIDS for the poorest families represented 82 percent of their annual revenue compared with 20 percent for the richest.

Access to antiretroviral therapy has dramatically improved the economic and social outlook of households, communities, and countries, besides saving the lives of those living with HIV.

A Generation of Orphans

The AIDS epidemic mainly affects adults but it also leaves behind many children without a mother, a father, or both. UNAIDS estimated that there are over fifteen million AIDS orphans in the world, 80 percent of whom are in Africa. They are often adopted by the extended family. Recent research in seven African countries describes the heavy burden these orphans represent for their families, and especially their grandparents, most often the grandmother. It is common for women to raise orphans, whether they have lost their mother, father, or both. The hardships of caring for orphans are particularly great for single-parent families headed by older women, usually grandmothers who take charge of orphans and vulnerable children and educate them when their own children fall ill or die. They had not expected to be parents for

Recent research in seven African countries describes the heavy burden these orphans represent for their families, and especially their grandparents, most often the grandmother. It is common for women to raise orphans, whether they have lost their mother, father, or both. The hardships of caring for orphans are particularly great for single-parent families headed by older women, usually grandmothers who take charge of orphans and vulnerable children and educate them when their own children fall ill or die. They had not expected to be parents for two generations!

two generations! Grandmothers raise almost 40 percent of orphans in Tanzania, 45 percent in Uganda, more than 50 percent in Kenya, and almost 60 percent in Namibia and Zimbabwe. In many poor countries older women are among the poorest and most marginalized members of society. Inequalities in employment, property, and inheritance laws, based on discrimination in favor of men, force many older women to continue to work until an advanced age. After the death of their husband elderly women often subsist with a pittance earned by hard work in nonstructured sectors. For example, in Uganda the FAO showed that widows worked two to four hours more per day to compensate the loss of revenue due to their husband's death. A dramatic rise in the number of orphans in Swaziland and Botswana has not only an economic cost, it also jeopardizes the future of a society composed in large part of orphans. Studies show that on average orphans are 10 to 15 percent less likely to go to school than non-orphans.

The most effective strategies to help orphans and other vulnerable children consist of offering them basic social protection, such as free access to medical care, schooling, or food aid. In 2010 only 15 to 20 percent of orphans in sub-Saharan Africa received any aid. Widows and grandmothers with children in charge should also have access to microcredit to help increase their revenue. In Kenya and Zambia fairer inheritance laws for widows have helped the situation of orphans.

Impact on Productivity and Services

In African countries with high HIV prevalence, the public and private sectors are confronted with increased costs due to absenteeism, reduced productivity, recruitment, training, and health care. In Southern Africa where the health sector chronically lacks personnel and is highly solicited by the epidemic, professionals are directly affected themselves. For example, Botswana lost 17 percent of its health personnel through AIDS between 1999 and 2005. Education has suffered particularly. Tanzania had to replace forty-five thousand experienced teachers over forty years old with newly recruited ones. The most economically affected sectors are those in which mobility of the male workers and their separation from their families is greatest, such as in agricultural plantations, mining, and transport, in which operating costs increased by 2 to 10 percent due to the impact of AIDS.

HIV also affects senior staff, such as in the banking sector in Southern Africa where absenteeism, recruitment, and training of new employees constituted a major additional expenditure due to AIDS. Wider access to antiretroviral therapy has reversed many of these economic impacts. Often, before governments offered antiretroviral treatment, several major companies in sub-Saharan Africa offered prevention and treatment to their employees living with HIV such as Heineken, Standard Chartered Bank, Anglo American, Debswana, and De Beers. Such programs usually paid off in terms of human lives and productivity. The South African public electricity company Eskom reported that its HIV programs resulted in lower infection levels among its personnel than the national average.

Financing the AIDS Response

Not only is the financial impact of the AIDS epidemic enormous, the sums needed to reverse it are also considerable. However, there is a significant payoff from investing in health in general.[6] In the case of AIDS, the positive impact of antiretroviral treatment is almost immediate for individuals, households, and communities, as illustrated earlier. In addition, if a well-targeted investment framework is used, necessary financing for prevention and treatment should decrease after an initial massive investment—primarily thanks to a gradual decline in new HIV infections, ultimately also reducing treatment costs.[7] The reality is that current levels of AIDS funding must at least be sustained for several decades to come in order to reach the point where they can be reduced without leading to a resurgence of new infections and deaths. This will require continued international funding to support the poorest countries with a heavy AIDS burden. According to UNAIDS, the financial needs for AIDS programs in low- and middle-income countries for 2015 are of the order of twenty-two billion dollars, whereas the funds available were around 15.9 billion in 2012. Global financing for the fight against AIDS increased

Where is the money coming from? Contrary to popular belief not all the funding of the fight against AIDS comes from the European, American, or Japanese taxpayer, but increasingly from the countries most affected, which in 2012 contributed just over 50 percent of expenditure—mostly from Nigeria, South Africa, and India.

from a few hundred thousand dollars in 2000 to approximately fifteen billion dollars in 2013. This has enabled AIDS programs to expand, both for prevention and treatment, resulting in millions of lives saved.

Where is the money coming from? Contrary to popular belief not all the funding of the fight against AIDS comes from the European, American, or Japanese taxpayer, but increasingly from the countries most affected, which in 2012 contributed just over 50 percent of expenditure— mostly from Nigeria, South Africa, and India. However, the reality is also that the financial burden of the AIDS response in many low-income African countries is enormous, and cannot be sustained by these state budgets alone. For example, a country such as Zambia would have to spend 3 to 4 percent of its annual GDP just on HIV treatment and prevention by 2030, which would be exorbitant for the state budget.[8] Today sub-Saharan African AIDS programs depend on international aid for almost three-quarters of their financing, and in some countries treatment of nearly all patients is paid for by international sources. In general, Latin America, Eastern Europe, and most of Asia depend little on international aid for their AIDS response. The United States is by far the greatest donor to the AIDS struggle worldwide, providing nearly 60 percent of the international contributions in 2012, including bilateral as well as multilateral aid. It is followed by the United Kingdom, France, Germany, and Japan. The Bill & Melinda Gates Foundationis a major private contributor, not only through its research and national programs, but also as a supporter of the Global Fund.

By far the two largest financing mechanisms for the global AIDS response are the Global Fund and PEPFAR, which is also the main

> The AIDS movement has generated a new type of multilateral financing mechanism in the Global Fund, which is now firmly established alongside traditional bilateral and multilateral funding. The GAVI Alliance, formerly the Global Alliance for Vaccines and Immunisation, is the other large financing institution operating along similar lines.

donor to the Global Fund. Their income depends largely on decisions by governments and parliaments, beginning in the U.S. Congress where there has been strong bipartisan support for global AIDS efforts, resulting in disbursement by PEPFAR of over fifty billion dollars by 2013 since its start in 2004, including nine billion dollars for the Global Fund. After some decline in funding, the replenishment conference in 2013 raised twelve billion dollars for 2014 to 2016 thanks to the strong leadership of Mark Dybul, who was also the U.S. global AIDS coordinator under President G. W. Bush.

The AIDS movement has generated a new type of multilateral financing mechanism in the Global Fund, which is now firmly established alongside traditional bilateral and multilateral funding. The GAVI Alliance, formerly the Global Alliance for Vaccines and Immunisation, is the other large financing institution operating along similar lines. The Fund's hallmarks are country-driven proposals, technical scrutiny of proposals, results-based disbursements, and great transparency of its operations and finances. The exemplary transparency of the Global Fund is dramatically illustrated by the detailed publication of cases of corruption among some of its grantees, and the action taken to recuperate missing funds. Corruption in the health sector is a worldwide phenomenon, including in high-income countries,[9] and among the 140 countries benefiting from the Global Fund there are twenty-three of the twenty-five worst in terms of corruption in Transparency International's Corruption Perceptions Index—though western and Japanese providers of commodities were involved as well in some corruption cases.

Tough Choices

There are a number of debates on resource allocation related to HIV/ AIDS, mainly concerning the rationale for investing massively in HIV as compared to other health issues, and on the relative importance of prevention and treatment.

According to the Global Burden of Disease 2010 study, HIV/AIDS ranks fifth and sixth respectively as the disease burden and cause of death globally, while ranking as the second cause of death and second cause of health loss in sub-Saharan Africa.[10] In Southern and some East African countries, HIV infection is by far the major cause of mortality and morbidity. Furthermore, its contagious nature with a continuing risk for further expansion of the epidemic, the risk of societal destabilization, and, crucially important for resource allocation in public health, the availability of highly cost-effective interventions, all amply justify national and international investments in the AIDS response. There has been criticism that AIDS programs have been relatively overfunded, as compared to other communicable and chronic diseases, or health services in general. This is probably the case in some countries with very low levels of HIV infection. It is correct that in many, if not most, countries health is indeed underfunded and governments have not honored their commitments to spending on health. For example, the 2001 Abuja Declaration called for African governments to spend 15 percent of their budget on health, but only a few countries have reached this level of funding. The real question therefore is not whether AIDS is overfunded, but how to also increase funding for other health issues and services.

The real question therefore is not whether AIDS is overfunded, but how to also increase funding for other health issues and services.

Whereas budgetary decision making should be based as much as possible on evidence, such as burden of disease and the return on investment of programs and interventions, it is primarily a political process reflecting power relations in a given society. In some countries the influence of civil society and business interests can be significant. The risk of national and international decision making is that the needs of smaller specific populations that are highly affected by HIV are neglected because they are stigmatized or in illegal situations. This not only leads to increased discrimination of such communities, but may also jeopardize overall AIDS efforts.

A collateral benefit of the AIDS movement has been a major boost in international funding for two long-neglected diseases—malaria and tuberculosis—through the Global Fund, financing for which is primarily driven by AIDS concerns. Together with the president's Malaria Initiative, the Global Fund now accounts for most international funding for these three infections.

Resource allocation within AIDS programs has been a longstanding controversial issue, in particular concerning treatment versus prevention and various prevention activities. Years of resistance by donor agencies, public health experts, and ministries of health to the introduction of antiretroviral treatment came to a definite end around the beginning of the new millennium. With the demonstration that antiretroviral treatment has a preventive benefit, the schism should come to an end—though it seems that the pendulum has swung too much to the treatment side, resulting in gross neglect of prevention programs. Although calls for a silver bullet for HIV prevention continue—the latest being "test and treat"—global consensus is now in favor of combination prevention, adapted to each micro-epidemic.[11] The question is now more about increased efficiency in any intervention and the relative weight of treatment and primary prevention as part of combination prevention (see chapter 6).

Components of combination prevention and their cost depend heavily on context, such as HIV incidence and modes of transmission, as discussed in the previous chapter. This makes estimates of global needs or comparisons of national expenditures on prevention not always useful to assess their potential impact on HIV spread. More refined financing models are needed at national and local level. With nearly two decades

Costs of antiretroviral therapy have evolved considerably as a result of lower prices of pharmaceuticals, but also vary widely between and within countries, usually due to management issues rather than the price of drugs.

of experience of large scale HIV interventions, it is clear that major gains in efficiency can be made in a number of critical AIDS program areas. Costs of interventions vary considerably depending on the local and economic context as well as the extent of the infection. The cost per DALY[12] averted was estimated in 2009[13] at between sixty-seven dollars and one hundred twelve dollars for HIV testing and counseling, three hundred eighty dollars to five hundred thirty dollars for sex education in schools, one hundred seventy-six dollars to two hundred ninety-two dollars for male circumcision in Southern Africa, and less than one hundred dollars for harm reduction programs for drug users. It varied from thirty-four dollars to three hundred ten dollars for the prevention of mother-to-child transmission, in Africa and Asia respectively. Even within the same country there may be enormous variations in cost and efficiency of HIV interventions. Thus in Russia testing and counseling can cost a few dollars per person, or forty times more. Only some of these wide differences in cost can be explained by economies of scale, and it seems that great inefficiencies in program implementation and even corruption may also account for the variations.

Costs of antiretroviral therapy have evolved considerably as a result of lower prices of pharmaceuticals (chapter 5), but also vary widely between and within countries, usually due to management issues rather than the price of drugs. For a long time discussions on access to antiretrovirals were centered purely on the cost of medication. Today it is clear that clinical staff costs and administration, laboratory tests, hospitalization, treatment of opportunistic infections and diseases related to HIV, and chronic anti-retroviral therapy cost at least twice as much as the antiretrovirals—in addition to patient costs for transport, extra nutritional requirements, and loss of income while attending clinics. These factors also influence the cost effectiveness of antiretroviral treatment. Thus in India[14] the cost of antiretroviral treatment is much lower if adherence is improved and if the cost of treatment for those living below the poverty threshold is covered. If in addition prevention, such as promotion of condom use, is linked to antiretroviral treatment the cost per life saved can be reduced even further. Increasing management efficiency and lowering costs of antiretroviral treatment as much as possible without compromising quality should be a priority for each country and HIV service, so that the maximum number of people can benefit. Increasing use of results-based disbursements by the Global Fund should be a major incentive for these efficiency gains.

How, and for what, are AIDS budgets spent? It is very variable, just like the epidemiological and administrative context of different countries. For example, in Eastern Europe and Central Asia, where most people infected with HIV are injecting drug users, AIDS budgets are mainly used for treatment or administrative costs, with a clear neglect of HIV prevention, in particular harm reduction programs. Similarly, in much of sub-Saharan Africa HIV prevention is insufficiently funded, as illustrated by Malawi, where only 11 percent of the AIDS budget was allocated for prevention in 2011. In heavily affected Lesotho,[15] in 2006 and 2007 only 10 percent of AIDS expenditure was for prevention, 33 percent for treatment and care, 24 percent for administration of programs, and 13 percent for supporting orphans. Worldwide in 2009 treatment and care programs received 56 percent of all available finance, and prevention just 20 percent. Seventy-one countries depended on international financing for more than half their prevention activities. In addition, prevention resources may not be attributed to where most new infections can be averted. In Botswana, for example, prevention funding focuses on mother-to-child transmission, whereas sexual transmission causes the overwhelming majority of new infections. In Latin America, for ideological and political reasons, most countries hardly finance prevention for gay communities, except for Mexico, Peru, and Brazil.

Future Challenges for HIV Financing

National and worldwide mobilization of funds for AIDS is an unprecedented achievement in international development, but the main challenge now is to sustain resources at a level that can bring the epidemic under control while keeping the over thirty-five million people living with HIV alive with a normal life expectancy. Despite a successful replenishment of twelve billion dollars for three years for the Global Fund in 2013 and continued commitment of the U.S. Administration and Congress, future funding for AIDS is fragile and uncertain. International assistance is for a major part a function of the health of the economies of donor countries, and recent years have seen an overall leveling of development assistance for health after tremendous growth at the beginning of the millennium.

The fiscal liability of the commitment to lifelong antiretroviral treatment is substantial, and may be beyond the capacity of some of the worst affected African countries. Hecht and colleagues[16] of aids2031 estimated that financial needs for AIDS programs will continue to increase over the next twenty years at a rate of two or three times more than today. Domestic financing will be pivotal in the long term: the accelerating economic growth of countries in Asia and Africa should lead to higher fiscal revenues, which can and should be used for health programs in addition to much-needed investments in infrastructure, education, and efficiency. It is likely that middle-income countries with a low burden of HIV will be able to cope fiscally, that low-income countries with a high burden (basically all in Africa) will remain reliant on international assistance for much of their AIDS response, and that middle-income countries with a high burden, such as those in Southern Africa, will probably require a mixture of domestic and international funding for AIDS years to come. Both PEPFAR and the Global Fund are now requesting domestic financing matching for between 5 and 60 percent of their grants.

A recurrent challenge and dilemma is prevention funding for stigmatized groups at high risk for HIV infection. They are often neglected by national AIDS programs in middle-income countries, which can afford such programs but opt not to do so for ideological reasons.

A recurrent challenge and dilemma is prevention funding for stigmatized groups at high risk for HIV infection. They are often neglected by national AIDS programs in middle-income countries, which can afford such programs but opt not to do so for ideological reasons. Diplomatic and technical pressure from the international community and institutions can sometimes induce policy change, but external support to NGOs working with neglected vulnerable populations should continue. There is the moral imperative to assist discriminated populations at risk of a deadly infection, but there is also the risk of wider HIV spread as a result of absent or ineffective prevention programs. Whereas most middle-income countries are financially able to manage their epidemic, there is an urgent need for a paradigm shift, ensuring that prevention programs and treatment services are fully accessible to marginal populations. Without such a paradigm shift, the end of AIDS will remain empty rhetoric.

"Innovative financing" is one of the buzz words in international development today, but there are very few concrete examples of such innovation—possibly because the options are quite limited. Examples in the AIDS arena include the AIDS levy in Zimbabwe, taxes on alcohol, social health insurance in Rwanda and Thailand, corporate AIDS programs, and airline taxes to fund UNITAID, which has played an innovative role in providing low cost antiretrovirals and other medicines.

There is a long-lasting need for a concerted global effort to sustain AIDS funding, besides institutionalizing the AIDS response in mainstream services wherever possible where not detrimental to the response. Serious attention must be paid to increasing the efficiency of prevention and treatment programs. It is not yet clear how to resolve the monumental long-term fiscal liabilities, and research in this area is only in its infancy. Sustaining global and national AIDS funding will require the provision of new epidemiological, economic, and developmental evidence[17]—not just rebranding or optimistic slogans. In the end only a significant fall in new infections will enable AIDS mortality to be reduced to low levels, and make the monetary costs of AIDS sustainable and affordable for every community.

8

PROMINENCE OF HUMAN RIGHTS

THE THIRD EPIDEMIC

I n 1987, from what was still an epidemic of unknown extent, Jonathan Mann, then-director of the WHO Special Programme on AIDS,[1] observed that for analytic purposes it was useful to consider AIDS as three distinct yet intertwined global epidemics. The first was the epidemic of HIV infection itself. The second, inexorably following the first but with a delay of several years, was the epidemic of AIDS. Unlike most infectious diseases, such as measles or yellow fever, which develop days or weeks after infection, AIDS may not occur until years or even decades after the initial infection. Finally, the third epidemic, of social, cultural, economic, and political reaction to AIDS, was worldwide and as central to the global challenge as the disease itself. Mann claimed that violation of human rights was the foundation of the AIDS epidemic. However, the reality is probably more complex, with no single element able to explain the epidemic spread of HIV, which is as much influenced by social, economic, and cultural contexts—not to mention sex drive.

The first decade of the AIDS epidemic was marked by the efforts of many states to control, by legal means or regulations, persons or groups affected by HIV. More than a hundred countries imposed laws one after the other.[2] When there is no remedy for a partly invisible, lethal infection governments turn to the law. Its strong association with stigmatization contributes largely to the special nature of AIDS. Thus in 1991 twelve countries ordered people living with HIV to be placed under surveillance. Seventeen imposed medical examination, isolation, detention, and compulsory treatment of people with the infection even though at the time there was no effective treatment. Countries like the Soviet Union or Bulgaria tested 30 to 40 percent of their total population. Fifteen countries imposed HIV testing for specific categories as varied as soldiers, pregnant women, prisoners, foreign students, refugees, immigrants, foreign residents, and patients with sexually transmitted diseases. Thirty countries soon classified HIV as a sexually transmitted disease, thus giving health authorities the possibility of taking measures to limit individual rights, notably restricting people with HIV from certain employments or international travel. An emblematic case was that of Hans-Paul Verhoef, a Dutch educator and gay activist detained in the United States in 1989 because he represented a "serious threat" for public health by trying to attend an AIDS conference: customs found the antiretroviral AZT in his bags. Verhoef admitted to having AIDS and died soon after.

These emergency public health measures reinforced stigmatization of people living with HIV and those who risked being infected. Practices such as compulsory screening of high-risk groups produced both additional stigmatization of these groups and a false sense of security in those who did not consider themselves to be concerned. At the beginning of the 1980s the term "4Hs" was used to characterize high-risk populations: homosexuals, hemophiliacs, heroin users, and Haitians. A whole population was suddenly associated with a lethal disease.

Faced with increasing AIDS-related discrimination worldwide Jonathan Mann and Daniel Tarantola placed human rights at the center of the fight against AIDS. In 1989 they organized, with the UN Centre for Human Rights, the first International Consultation on HIV/AIDS and Human Rights. The principles of public health for the prevention of discrimination associated with HIV were reaffirmed, as well as promotion and protection of human rights. This position was reinforced in resolutions of the UN General Assembly in 1990 and 1991. In May 1992 the World Health Assembly emphasized the relationship between public health and protection of the rights of those infected with HIV. Mann and Tarantola left WHO at the beginning of the 1990s and continued, with

Sofia Gruskin, to further the relationship between human rights and public health at Harvard University. Partly as a result of the advocacy of WHO and UNAIDS many countries promulgated laws to protect the rights of people with HIV in the 1990s.[3] In 2010 70 percent of countries had laws and regulations to guarantee the right to employment, education, private life, and confidentiality, as well as to information, treatment, and support for people living with HIV.

THE BIG SCARE

Stigmatization is the disapproval of an individual or a group because they are different in the eyes of other members of society. It tends to associate AIDS with marginalized "deviant" behavior such as prostitution, drug use, and particularly homosexuality. Discrimination is the "operational" result of stigmatization. As defined by UNAIDS[4] "discrimination refers to any form of distinction, exclusion or restriction affecting a person, usually, but not only, by virtue of an inherent personal characteristic, irrespective of whether or not there is any justification for these measures." In the case of HIV discrimination is defined as "Any measure entailing an arbitrary distinction among persons depending on their confirmed or suspected HIV serostatus or state of health."

AIDS as a Social Disease

At the very beginning of the epidemic fear of AIDS was understandable as we did not fully understand the mechanisms of transmission of this fatal disease. This type of societal reaction was not new. Throughout history, stigma and infection have often been associated, from the medieval plague to tuberculosis, leprosy, and syphilis. Tuberculosis was a shameful disease, provoking genuine fear of contagion and stigmatization of the poor. Syphilis and certain cancers or mental illnesses provoked widespread fear and provoked social discrimination. Susan Sontag stated in her 1989 book *AIDS and Its Metaphors* that nothing is more punitive than giving moral significance to a disease.[5] Using the same logic, the patient,

> As Michel Foucault emphasized, sexual behavior has often been either an ethical issue or "a domain of moral experience." The definition of the disease as a sanction, a moral punishment, means holding people responsible and guilty for their infection.

as an example of the ills and contradictions of society, becomes the scapegoat. In his *History of Madness*, Michel Foucault[6] showed, for example, the difference between the social treatment of leprosy, characterized by exclusion, and that of the plague, a sort of inclusion through the process of quarantine even in the heart of cities. The AIDS pandemic, by its global character, has given rise to a wide diversity of cultural interpretations. For Mirko Grmek[7] AIDS is a metaphorical disease: "with its links to sex, drugs, blood, and informatics, and with the sophistication of its evolution and of its strategy for spreading itself, AIDS expresses our era."

AIDS is often presented as a punitive disease sanctioning sexual promiscuity. As Michel Foucault emphasized,[8] sexual behavior has often been either an ethical issue or "a domain of moral experience." The definition of the disease as a sanction, a moral punishment, means holding people responsible and guilty for their infection. In some traditional cultures in Africa, fatal diseases in young adults are considered punishment for transgression of taboos meted out by supernatural powers. AIDS is therefore the consequence of not respecting social norms and provokes rejection and condemnation.

The fear of contagion remains a powerful driver of discrimination in spite of scientific clarification of modes of transmission. Beliefs are still very much alive that contamination can happen invisibly simply by contact with bodily fluids or objects soiled by such fluids. These beliefs isolate people with HIV and double their suffering. Referring to his magisterial novel *The Plague*, Albert Camus said, "I wish to express, by means of the plague, the feeling of suffocation from which we all suffered and the atmosphere of threat and exile in which we lived."[9] The terminology used with reference to AIDS also contributes to reinforcing these stereotypes.[10] In nearly all cultures there are contemptuous expressions to describe people living with HIV. For example, in Tanzania a person with HIV is often called "maiti inayotembea" ("walking corpse") or "marehemu mtaxajiwa" ("about to die"). People rarely talk about AIDS openly, preferring to use an expression such as "that disease we've heard of."

An Epidemic Nurtured by Injustices

Thirty years after its appearance, we now know how HIV is transmitted and sheer panic no longer has any place. But despite a fair understanding of AIDS in most societies false ideas about its spread persist and continue to encourage stigmatization and discrimination. In contrast to what many had hoped for when antiretroviral therapy became widely available, HIV infection was not "normalized" and society's view of people with HIV remains pejorative.

Often HIV infection is a motive for pre-existing discrimination.[11] Thus foreigners or immigrants are suspected of having introduced the virus and contaminated the healthy population. Prostitutes are stigmatized as a vector of infection. For example, drug use and prostitution are seen as social evils in Vietnam and China, and infected people as perpetrators of antisocial behavior. In Thailand in 2003 the war against drugs was more a war against drug users and led to the extrajudicial execution of more than two thousand people. In Russia and parts of the United States the possession of unused syringes is considered a criminal offense. In many countries, particularly in Eastern Europe and Central Asia, drug users do not have equal access to antiretrovirals. In most Asian countries, like Vietnam and Cambodia, drug addicts can be forced into detention centers for years.

In some countries women are seen as responsible for the spread of HIV. Women often learn of their HIV infection before their partner when attending an antenatal clinic, and may be blamed for bringing the infection into the couple. Women with HIV are often ill treated and abandoned by their husbands, although it is often he who was at the origin of their infection. Violence toward women is widespread[12] and

> Homophobia is one of the most common forms of structural discrimination. Consensual sex between adults of the same sex is forbidden in over seventy countries. Attacks against men suspected of homosexuality are common in many parts of the world, including Europe and the United States. They are sometimes related to AIDS.

may be nurtured by ancient social and cultural concepts that make it quite acceptable within a society, as much among the women as the men. Many studies throughout the world confirm a link between violence against women and HIV.[13] Thus women with HIV are more frequently victims of violence, and women suffering violence are more likely to be infected with HIV. In national demographic and health studies on intimate partner violence, between 10 and 69 percent of women suffered physical violence at least once in their life from a male partner. In India a study showed that men who have extramarital sex are six times more likely to inflict sexual violence on their wives than other men.[14] Female victims of violence and male domination use condoms less frequently than other women. It is estimated that about one third of the first sexual relations in South African women are forced.

Homophobia is one of the most common forms of structural discrimination. Consensual sex between adults of the same sex is forbidden in over seventy countries.[15] Attacks against men suspected of homosexuality are common in many parts of the world, including Europe and the United States. They are sometimes related to AIDS. It is a very long and revolting list. For example, in Senegal local AIDS activists accused of being gay were arrested when they organized a meeting on HIV prevention. In Malawi a male homosexual couple was condemned to fourteen years in prison before being reprieved by the president under international pressure. In Burundi several homosexual men were beaten to death. In Uganda gay activist David Kato, whose name was published by a magazine calling for his death, was murdered in the midst of a homophobic campaign, and parliament approved a law severely punishing homosexuality and even punishing the lack of denouncing homosexual activity. In Central America dozens of homosexual men engaged in human rights activities have been murdered. In spite of antidiscrimination laws in some countries, there are probably thousands of homophobic murders per year globally. In China homosexuality is not illegal but in practice there is persecution. In Eastern Europe, Russia, and Central Asia aggressive homophobia is widespread and discrimination and violence are common, including torture and murder by police forces. Even senior political leaders speak with virulence against homosexuality, and the Russian parliament voted a severe law against homosexuality and even information about it. Homophobia and illegality of homosexuality make HIV prevention and treatment programs very difficult, so this discrimination makes men who have sex with men even more vulnerable to infection.

DISCRIMINATION

HIV-related discrimination can be found in numerous contexts, including the family, the local community, the workplace, and health services. Among the most common are violations of data protection, especially results of HIV testing. Discrimination related to HIV is reported from most countries. For example, in China[16] in 2009 42 percent of people living with HIV experienced one or several forms of discrimination. Thirty percent reported their serostatus disclosed without their permission, 12 percent were refused medical care, 35 percent experienced discrimination by employers or colleagues—all this despite progressive antidiscrimination laws. Among those with children 9 percent were forced to withdraw their children from school and 10 percent of HIV-positive women were forced to terminate pregnancy.

The Workplace

The workplace is a common place for HIV-related discrimination. A study in France showed that discrimination in the workplace was widespread in spite of mass campaigns against it. It found that discrimination at recruitment was common; 33 percent of people living with HIV in 2005 and 27 percent in 2008 encountered discrimination in the workplace from ostracism to insults and psychological harassment, and that 31 percent had lost their employment. In severely affected countries, especially in industries in which employees can benefit from health insurance, HIV testing at recruitment is widespread, with rejection of candidates who test positive. This shows the need to ensure that companies enforce active antidiscrimination policies.

Health Services

Although this should be the last place where it happens, discrimination in the health care environment is common, not only in low-income countries. A study in 2009 in the United Kingdom[17] revealed that 47 percent of people with HIV had suffered infringement of their rights. Seventeen percent were refused care because of their infection status and 31 percent had an unconstructive relationship with their care provider. A study by the Moroccan Association for the Fight against AIDS in 2009 showed that discrimination in the health services remained very serious, with 40 percent of people with HIV experiencing it at least once and 11 percent in the previous twelve months. In a study in four Asian countries[18] 54 percent of people with HIV stated having encountered various forms of discrimination in the health sector, from refusal of admission to a health center to refusal or delay of medical care. It is hard to understand how medical personnel place their moral beliefs and prejudices above their duty to care and medical ethics. Zero tolerance for such behavior should be the norm in every health care setting.

Restrictions to Freedom of Movement

Another common form of HIV-related discrimination is the right of entry to a country. Seventy-four states impose restrictions to entry or residency for people living with HIV, including Russia, Egypt, Iraq, Singapore, and Poland. Twenty-four expel people if HIV infection is detected. The reasons given concern the risk of transmission to the local population or the cost of treatment. Some states insist on a declaration of noninfection before admission while others require a negative HIV test. Since 2010 people with HIV can enter the United States and China, from which they were banned before. Some countries with a strong track record on human rights, such as Australia and Canada, also have restrictions for permanent residence. This is another illustration that AIDS in not a disease like any other, although untreated tuberculosis also often leads to a ban on entry. These regulations are essentially political.

Collateral Human Rights Benefits of AIDS

The AIDS response has also had a positive impact on some pre-existing human rights problems. Paradoxically, the status of homosexual men, the group most affected by HIV, has become much more mainstream in society in many countries. So a deadly infection that threatened to destroy a community actually contributed to the resilience and emancipation of that community. This has been the case in North America, Western Europe, and some of Latin America, where the public at large and the media have developed a greater appreciation of sexual diversity, in particular gay culture. In France, for example, there has been a steady increase over thirty years in the opinion that homosexuality is an acceptable way to live one's life, from 24 percent in 1973 to 78 percent in 2006. Let us not forget that homosexuality was considered a mental illness until the 1980s in numerous countries, and as recently as 1993 by the World Health Organization.

These changes in public opinion have led to a legal framework that guarantees equal rights regardless of sexual orientation, including the right to marriage. This has been particularly the case in Western Europe, and in some American states and Canada, but also in South Africa, whereas in other countries, such as Nigeria and Uganda, legal discrimination of homosexuality has worsened. In 2008 Mexico, where men who have sex with men are by far the most affected by HIV, introduced several laws against discrimination on the grounds of sexual orientation. Fiji abolished its laws on homosexual relations by replacing its penal code. Nepal recognized the rights of sexual minorities in its new constitution.

> The AIDS movement has also given a public voice to those who had no voice, and brought people affected by the epidemic to the decision table. This was a first in public health, which has traditionally been the domain of experts and administrators.

That progress in this sensitive area can be one step forward and two steps back is illustrated by the saga around Section 377 of the penal code in India—a law criminalizing same-sex relations going back to British colonial times and still active in several Commonwealth countries, such as in the Caribbean. In 2009 the New Delhi High Court overturned Section 377, only to be overruled by the Supreme Court in 2013 with the argument that only new legislation can change the law. Whereas a law does not change prejudice and stigma, a protective legal framework is a major step for the full enjoyment of all rights by sexual minorities, and also to encourage open and effective HIV prevention and treatment.

The AIDS response pioneered access to lifesaving treatment with medicines still under patent through a change in the TRIPS rules on intellectual property, as well as a change in pharmaceutical companies' practices and the emergence of the Indian pharmaceutical industry, resulting in access to generic antiretroviral treatment (see chapter 5). This may set a precedent for access to treatment for other diseases in environments with poor resources.[19]

The AIDS movement has also given a public voice to those who had no voice, and brought people affected by the epidemic to the decision table. This was a first in public health, which has traditionally been the domain of experts and administrators. Today representatives of nongovernmental and community-based organizations, and of groups of people living with HIV, participate in national AIDS programs and discuss technical, budgetary, and political priorities. They are also members of the Programme Coordinating Board of UNAIDS and the Board of the Global Fund, where they are co-responsible for governance decisions. The involvement of people living with HIV has introduced a new model for accountability, including publicly revealing discussions held behind closed doors, and by publishing independent performance reports on institutions, countries, and companies.[20]

HOW TO COUNTER DISCRIMINATION

There was great hope that the wide availability of antiretroviral treatment would dispel HIV-related stigma and that AIDS would be seen as an "ordinary" disease. Unfortunately this turned out not to be the case, and countering stigma and discrimination requires as much an evidence-informed programmatic approach as HIV prevention. A first and essential step is the recognition that every AIDS program needs an antidiscrimination component in order to be fully effective—not just to promote human rights. HIV prevention and treatment programs suffer in a context of stigma and discrimination, as shown in a UNAIDS report that documented that HIV rates are higher in the presence of purely repressive drug policies.

It is the role of the state to guarantee such rights and introduce public health programs designed for maximum impact on people's health; advocacy for legal change and supportive laws will remain necessary. The Global Commission on HIV and the Law provides practical examples of legislative work for HIV support.[21] Legal action whenever there are violations of human rights and instances of HIV-related discrimination is an important way of furthering the agenda through jurisprudence, drawing public attention to injustices. International Guideline 5 of the UN High Commission for Human Rights is quite clear:[22]

> States should enact or strengthen anti-discrimination and other protective laws that protect vulnerable groups, people living with HIV and people with disabilities from discrimination in both the public and private sectors, ensure privacy and confidentiality and ethics in research involving human subjects, emphasize education and conciliation, and provide for speedy and effective administrative and civil remedies.

> With the increasing adoption of antiretroviral therapy as the main, if not the only, response to AIDS, there seems to be a growing underappreciation of the need to promote human rights and counter stigma and discrimination as part of every AIDS program. This would greatly undermine the AIDS response.

Several simultaneous approaches are needed to influence HIV-related attitudes and norms, including awareness campaigns, programs in the workplace and in schools, statements by celebrities, activism, and legal change and enforcement. In the end it is often an issue of leadership by those in charge of AIDS programs, as well as by societal, business, religious, and media leaders. A good example of a comprehensive approach was in Switzerland, which integrated innovative campaigns against discrimination of seropositive people into its regular HIV prevention and treatment programs. This resulted in better acceptance of people living with HIV, though discrimination has not entirely disappeared.

The workplace provides precious opportunities for combating HIV-related stigma and discrimination, and there are now outstanding examples of companies and institutions that have embraced "positive action" with people living with HIV, from Levi Strauss in San Francisco to companies operating in Africa like Standard Chartered Bank and Heineken Breweries, and UN Plus, the group of HIV-positive UN employees. Creating an environment in which people living with HIV can openly live, work, speak out, and give a human face to a largely hidden epidemic, is one of the best foundations for positive change for people living with HIV.

With the increasing adoption of antiretroviral therapy as the main, if not the only, response to AIDS, there seems to be a growing under-appreciation of the need to promote human rights and counter stigma and discrimination as part of every AIDS program. This would greatly undermine the AIDS response. First, there is no significant decrease in stigma and discrimination, undermining the rights of people living with HIV as well as the effectiveness of and access to prevention and treatment. Second, discriminatory and counterproductive legislative initiatives continue to be launched and sometimes adopted by parliaments. Thus more than fifteen African states introduced penal laws specific to HIV. In general, these laws are vague, with overextensive provisions sanctioning transmission. For example, in Sierra Leone the law specifically criminalizes seropositive mothers who transmit HIV to their children during pregnancy, labor, or breastfeeding. Certain of these laws could be applied disproportionately and abusively against women, who often discover their infection before their husband and have less means to defend themselves in court. Obviously, if one person deliberately infects someone through unprotected sex it is morally and, depending on the circumstances and the country, judicially unacceptable, in particular in the case of coercion or rape.

According to South African High Court Justice Edwin Cameron[23] criminalization of HIV infection increases stigmatization by sending a message that we must find the guilty party. But in most cases HIV spreads through consensual sexual relations between people who do not know they are infected.

9

THE LONG-TERM VIEW

When AIDS emerged in 1981, and throughout the 1980s, we implicitly believed that it would be a short-lived crisis. The question of when it would end was rarely discussed and for more than two decades there was essentially no consideration that HIV infection might be a long-term epidemic. For two decades a vaccine was promised in the next five years. Everything we have learned about the virus, what drives its spread and how to control it, tell us that HIV will be with us for a long time—decades, if not generations, depending on when an effective vaccine will be available. Even if by some miracle its transmission ceased today, the world would still have more than thirty-five million people living with HIV who at some point will all need antiretroviral treatment for decades requiring colossal budgets. In addition there will be millions of orphans. This is a disturbing reality, particularly in an era characterized by short termism[1] and at a time of great medical optimism that the end of the epidemic is a matter of a few years away. While intensifying current efforts to decrease mortality from HIV and reduce its spread to low endemic levels, AIDS programs and societies at large should shift the current paradigm of an emergency response to a long-term sustained effort.

REVISITING THE PREVENTION STRATEGY

There is no doubt that the number of new HIV infections is declining globally, but with over two million new infections in 2013 it is difficult to speak of success, and we are a long way from reducing incidence to very low levels, let alone elimination of HIV. In theory, if all currently available preventive measures are consistently applied to all those in need, the epidemic can be reduced to low levels in our lifetime. Some mathematical models have even predicted elimination of HIV transmission by as early as 2020[2] through testing and early treatment. However, assumptions of the real-life effectiveness of interventions used in these models are overoptimistic: the models generally fail to address the uneven distribution of infection in a population, with a cumulative patchwork of micro-epidemics occurring in groups at different risks of HIV.[3] The transmission and treatment dynamics in each micro-epidemic vary widely, with an overall decline in incidence possibly masking an increase in highly affected populations.

Several recent trends in various parts of the world are a major cause for concern, and may be the writing on the wall that the end of AIDS is not yet in sight, and that there is a need to reassess strategies. There is rising HIV incidence in Uganda, continuing high incidence in Swaziland in spite of high antiretroviral coverage, and epidemics among men who have sex with men in North America, Asia, and Europe in a context of good access to antiretrovirals. All these factors go against more favorable trends elsewhere, and require special attention. In addition new high-risk behaviors have appeared that expand the number of vulnerable people, such as injecting drug use in several African countries. Another critical factor for HIV spread is that the number of sexually active adolescents and young adults will be greater than ever before in history, particularly in sub-Saharan Africa, expanding the pool of susceptible individuals, even if they practice safer sex than the previous generation.

If prevention programs continue at the current pace, and even if they are intensified to pay more attention to key populations at risk and include antiretroviral treatment at early stages of infection, there will probably be a continued slow decline in the number of new infections, rather than a sudden collapse of the epidemic. According to modeling by the aids2031 Consortium, with a favorable scenario of funding and intensified programs, there would still be around one million new HIV infections globally by 2030, rather than elimination. Whereas these projections may be too pessimistic, they could also be optimistic. In South Africa, for example, at the peak of the epidemic in 1995 there were more than seven hundred thousand new HIV infections per year. Aids2031

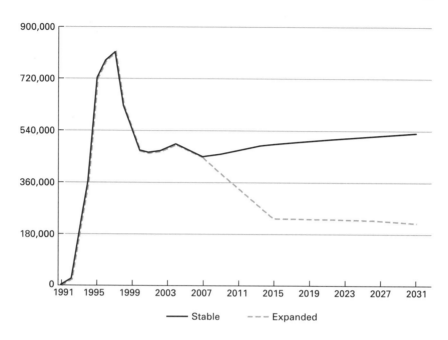

SOURCE: AIDS2031 WORKING GROUP PROJECTIONS.

FIGURE 9.1 NUMBER OF ANNUAL NEW HIV INFECTIONS IN ADULTS AGED FIFTEEN
TO FORTY-NINE IN SOUTH AFRICA FROM 1991 TO 2031.

projections suggested stabilization starting in 2010 as long as programs
continued to be pursued at the same level (figure 9.1). In the best case
scenario, there would still be one hundred fifty thousand to two hundred
thousand new infections per year for the next twenty years in a country
with over fifty-two million inhabitants in 2014. If antiretroviral treatment has a larger impact on transmission than assumed in the model,
the number would be lower, though not zero. Even with improved access
to antiretrovirals AIDS mortality will probably still remain high, up to
two hundred thousand per year.[4]

One of the great unknowns for the future of the HIV epidemic is
its evolution in Asia. Contrary to what we thought in the 1990s neither India nor China experienced an explosive generalized epidemic as
in sub-Saharan Africa. Thailand, Cambodia, and Burma experienced

low-grade generalized epidemics and succeeded in reducing infections in the general population, but transmission in high-risk populations continues at high rates. In Malaysia and Indonesia, where HIV was mainly associated with injecting drug use, sexual transmission is now becoming the main mode of transmission, though still at low levels. The next twenty years of HIV infection in Asia are largely unpredictable, given the major unknowns of how economic development and social change will affect sexual behavior, and the size and dynamics of various micro-epidemics. Major changes in sexual behavior have been documented in large Asian cities like Hanoi, Shanghai, or Taipei,[5] and in Japan: a greater expression of sexual diversity among both men and women may make them more vulnerable to HIV infection. Changes in sexual lifestyles have also been observed in Britain, including larger numbers of heterosexual partners in women, and more same-sex partners.[6] In contrast, in some parts of the world or in sub-populations, social change could also lead to stricter sexual norms under the influence of conservative or fundamentalist movements.

The long-term approach to the HIV epidemic places reinvigorated prevention beside universal access to antiretroviral therapy at its core.[7] This will be essential to bring the current HIV pandemic down to low endemic levels over the next few decades in all populations concerned—not just the low-risk heterosexual population. The evidence that treatment will end the epidemic in the presence of high-risk sexual and injecting behavior is still very limited. Given the large number of uncertain operational parameters for providing lifelong treatment to tens of millions of people in a wide range of social and economic contexts, it

> The long-term approach to the HIV epidemic places reinvigorated prevention beside universal access to antiretroviral therapy at its core. This will be essential to bring the current HIV pandemic down to low endemic levels over the next few decades in all populations concerned—not just the low-risk heterosexual population.

will be very difficult to achieve high levels of lifelong antiretroviral treatment and adherence among all those in need.

This renewed effort in HIV prevention will require a strategic repositioning of national and international AIDS programs with a resolute adoption of combination prevention as discussed in chapter 6. Above all, relevant and effective combinations of interventions should be tailored to the needs of the various micro-epidemics. Resources must be focused on populations with high transmission, with regular adaptation when epidemic dynamics evolve.[8] HIV prevention must also make better use of new social media and communication technologies, such as the mobile telephone, which are playing an increasing role in sexual networking. Incentive-based behavioral interventions for HIV prevention such as cash transfers should also be more widely explored for their cost effectiveness.

The challenges for prevention are enormous in populations with continuing annual HIV incidence rates of 1 to 6 percent, as experienced in the general population in parts of Southern Africa and in some communities of men who have sex with men, sex workers, and drug users. It is likely that new prevention methods based on antiretrovirals, such as microbicides and oral pre-exposure prophylaxis (PrEP), will need to be part of combination prevention in such populations. Their user acceptability and cost will be major determinants whether they will be widely used. Any long-term approach to the HIV epidemic should aim at more than changing individual sexual behavior. It should also promote changes in social norms, especially those concerning sexual inequality, sexual minorities, and sex-based violence.

Eliminating HIV-Related Mortality

Spectacular progress has been achieved in access to antiretroviral treatment, far beyond the skepticism and cynicism of the mainstream public health and development experts in the 1990s (chapter 5). And yet in 2013 1.5 million people still died from HIV infection, most of them because they had either no access to antiretrovirals or were not aware of their infection. With WHO now recommending for both clinical and

Sub-Saharan Africa, with 11 percent of the world's population, 24 percent of the world's disease burden, and 68 percent of the world's HIV population, houses only 3 percent of the world's health personnel.

preventive reasons that treatment be initiated when CD4 counts are at or below five hundred cells per mm3, a majority of the over thirty-five million people living with HIV are now in need of antiretroviral treatment, as compared to around ten million in treatment in 2013.

Current and future needs for antiretroviral treatment are enormous, in particular in countries with weak health care services. How can we face this growing need when health services in poor countries suffer from a chronic lack of personnel and equipment, often aggravated by a drain of human resources to richer countries? Sub-Saharan Africa, with 11 percent of the world's population, 24 percent of the world's disease burden, and 68 percent of the world's HIV population, houses only 3 percent of the world's health personnel. This means that there is an imperative to develop more effective approaches to health care delivery, which would also be an opportunity to develop original affordable models for chronic care—a growing need across the world due to the rise in cardiovascular disease, cancer, diabetes, obesity, and dementia. Such new models include task shifting (see chapter 5) and integrating AIDS care in mainstream health and community services. For example, in Uganda antiretroviral treatment provided the same clinical benefits for patients whether provided in a health center or in the community, but a community service was much less costly for the patient, and perhaps improved adherence to the treatment. In Lesotho, entrusting patient care to nurses and trained counselors resulted in better follow-up and adherence than treatment provided by physicians in a hospital setting. In KwaZulu-Natal, the treatment of patients co-infected with tuberculosis and HIV benefited from the use of trained community auxiliaries. The simplification and standardization of laboratory tests, in particular for viral load, should also improve health care performance. The cumulative effect of optimization at every step of treatment should result in more people benefiting fully from antiretroviral treatment for the same budget, if not "more with less."[9]

In high-income countries cutting edge medicine takes care of the long-term complications of antiretroviral treatment, including accelerated ageing, metabolic, cardiovascular and other problems, and the long-term evolution of infection. But with over ten million people now on antiretrovirals in poor resource settings, how will their chronic clinical problems be managed? There is an urgent need to develop simplified and affordable clinical strategies for such chronic care, not only to enroll more people for antiretroviral treatment. As for regular antiretroviral treatment, the *how* of clinical management is at least as important as the *what*.

Resistance of HIV to antiretrovirals is unavoidable as fast mutating viruses such as HIV develop survival mechanisms, particularly when treatment adherence is imperfect or drug regimens are inappropriate. It is not clear how much of a clinical problem such resistance will be in the near or distant future. Consistent prescription of standardized drug regimens for first- and second-line antiretroviral therapy, combined with more widespread use of viral load testing at the point of care, and community, economic, and behavioral interventions to enhance adherence to treatment, should all contribute to minimize the development of resistance. They must be part of a long-term AIDS strategy. At the same time the high level of chronic infection, problems of long-term treatment, and the threat of large-scale resistance to antiretrovirals point to a continuing need to invest in research for new anti-HIV medicines.

Finance

As discussed in chapter 7, long-term costs for HIV prevention and treatment are significant. Unless there is a major technological advance the needs of middle- and low-income countries for fighting AIDS will increase to reach between nineteen and thirty-five billion dollars per year in 2031, which is two to three times more than today.[10] The financial liability of lifelong antiretroviral treatment for millions of people is substantial, and may be beyond the capacity of some low-income African countries with major epidemics, with such liabilities costing the equivalent of up to three times the annual GDP of countries such as Uganda and Swaziland.[11] In the short term, global and national financing of HIV programs seem solid, though with little room for expansion, particularly since the successful replenishment of the Global Fund in 2013 with twelve billion dollars for three years and continued commitment of the U.S. administration and Congress. However, long-term funding for AIDS is fragile and by definition uncertain, as is any public budget. As mentioned earlier, strategic choices for the HIV response over the next few years will not only have a decisive influence on the future trajectory of the epidemic, but also on the ultimate costs to society. A useful investment framework for AIDS was developed by UNAIDS, but it now requires further prioritization of activities and opportunities for improved efficiency.[12]

AIDS has generated new mechanisms for international financing in health, such as the Global Fund. At the same time, such global funding has basically been part of classic international assistance for development. It is not clear how development aid will evolve in the coming decades. How much will it be, and what form will it take? There seems to be a trend for development assistance to focus on global public goods like international security, financial stability, normative assistance, response to global warming, or control of major pandemics.[13] Even if the current favorable economic growth continues for the poorest and worst affected countries in sub-Saharan Africa, they will most likely continue to need external support for many years to come to confront AIDS.[14]

Sustained financing of the AIDS response will require more than repeating arguments of moral persuasion, societal impact of AIDS, good return on investment, and calls by celebrities. Ministers of finance will increasingly ask hard questions as to why the AIDS bill increases every year, what the results are, and why they should invest in AIDS activities instead of other health and social issues.

It is encouraging that middle-income countries are now paying for most of their AIDS response, resulting in a greater share of international financing for low-income countries.

Sustained financing of the AIDS response will require more than repeating arguments of moral persuasion, societal impact of AIDS, good return on investment, and calls by celebrities. Ministers of finance will increasingly ask hard questions as to why the AIDS bill increases every year, what the results are, and why they should invest in AIDS activities instead of other health and social issues. Besides resolute local and international leadership, it will require increased domestic public investments in low- and middle-income countries. This will include commitment to policy change and support of key affected populations, a revisited strategy for more effective HIV prevention, and better management of existing resources. It perhaps means a major "rebranding" of the response to AIDS.

Leadership

One of the main lessons of the global response to AIDS of the last thirty years has been that without political and community leadership there would have been no progress. Good leadership has changed the situation in countries, communities, businesses, religious institutions, and NGOs. Today there is less attention being paid to AIDS in the media and the occasional manifestations of interest are related to major international conferences or on World AIDS Day on December 1.

Even AIDS activism seems to have declined in many countries, possibly sparked by internal conflicts or due to weariness, lack of means, and perhaps wider access to treatment that has trivialized AIDS in many communities. There is a need for a new generation of activists to emphasize the need to continue to invest in the AIDS response, speak up for neglected and stigmatized communities, and hold governments and institutions accountable for their promises of action on AIDS. Without such activism, pressure on governments may be too weak to sustain commitments. Whereas for a decade AIDS was on the agenda of major global and regional bodies, such as the G8, this is no longer the

A new leadership is emerging among young people and may be less concentrated around individuals and media stars. It is vital that new leadership be institutionalized as part of a country's or community's mainstream development and health agenda. This is particularly important in countries with a high HIV burden, such as in Southern and Eastern Africa.

case, with the exception of the African Union, thanks to the advocacy of UNAIDS executive director Michel Sidibé.

A new leadership is emerging among young people and may be less concentrated around individuals and media stars. It is vital that new leadership be institutionalized as part of a country's or community's mainstream development and health agenda. This is particularly important in countries with a high HIV burden, such as in Southern and Eastern Africa, where AIDS should be an issue regularly debated in parliament by the representatives of the people and at government cabinet meetings. Funding should be a regular budget item.

Program Implementation

Now that numerous countries and institutions have considerable experience in HIV prevention and treatment, often on a large scale, a major challenge for the long-term approach to AIDS is improving program delivery. First, we can do better with current budgets, and thereby reach more people in need of prevention and treatment.[15] Second, the management of long-term chronic care requires a major overhaul to make it effective, sustainable, and affordable on a large scale.[16] Third, some of the failures of reaching marginalized and discriminated populations are not only due to policy obstacles but to poor management and service delivery. Improvement will require the best of public service rigor, NGO enthusiasm, and business world entrepreneurship and incentives. It will require a review of incentives and performance indicators, as well as internalizing results of experimentation and regular evaluation of work at all levels, with serious accountability to relevant stakeholders. None of this is specific for AIDS programs, but as it has done so often, the AIDS response could innovate in a way that is useful for other health programs and care services in general.

Research and Innovation

Much of our progress in the AIDS response is due to scientific discovery and innovation, with the introduction in 1996 of highly active antiretrovirals being the most spectacular game changer. Bringing this epidemic under control will require further research and innovation. The key biomedical research questions are the development of a vaccine, a cure, and new drugs. Considerable progress has been made in our basic virological and immunological understanding of HIV infection, providing a scientific basis for vaccine development, but only clinical trials in humans can actually demonstrate protection.[17] Only one such trial (RV144) in Thailand[18] with a combination of two different vaccines has shown modest protection (an efficacy of 26 to 31 percent), establishing proof of concept that protective immunity can be induced, and providing a boost for vaccine research. Even if the perspective of a vaccine remains distant, research is vital, as without a widely available effective vaccine, it is unlikely that the HIV epidemic can be ended.[19]

Similarly, on the basis of a few patients, there is now proof of concept that cure of HIV infection is possible, and much innovative research is

Bringing this epidemic under control will require further research and innovation. The key biomedical research questions are the development of a vaccine, a cure, and new drugs. Considerable progress has been made in our basic virological and immunological understanding of HIV infection, providing a scientific basis for vaccine development, but only clinical trials in humans can actually demonstrate protection.

being conducted. The ultimate goal is to develop a cure that can be used affordably on a large scale in resource-poor settings. The development of new antiretroviral drugs remains necessary to preempt and overcome resistance against existing antiretrovirals, and also to enhance patient acceptability for lifelong treatment through long-acting medication and a reduction in side effects. Finally, simple point of care diagnostics for monitoring antiretroviral therapy are increasingly needed as the duration of treatment increases.

Another critical area of research needed is the development and evaluation of HIV prevention, as detailed in chapter 6. This should include more research into behavioral and structural interventions. Even antiretroviral treatment has major behavioral components that require more research, notably how to improve adherence to medication. A third area of research is implementation and operational research. This is as important for the control of HIV infection as basic research, but is grossly underfunded. It should be linked to a more rigorous agenda of evaluation of real-life programs, with constant feedback to AIDS programs and practitioners. Finally, research on economic, financial, and political dimensions of a long-term AIDS response will be essential to inform decision makers in their funding policies and to design financial options for a sustained response.

The End?

The short history of AIDS has shown above all that when politics, science, and service delivery work in synergy, mountains can be moved to save lives across the globe. The world is now entering a new phase in the fight against AIDS: the armamentarium for prevention and treatment is more powerful than ever, and HIV incidence and mortality are declining in much of the world. At the same time there are the first signs of fragility with a rise in incidence in previously successful populations, while high infection rates continue to prevail in key vulnerable communities and regions. There may now be a narrow window of opportunity to capitalize on scientific advances and on political momentum to

> There may now be a narrow window of opportunity to capitalize on scientific advances and on political momentum to accelerate the positive trajectory toward reducing the global epidemic to low endemic levels.

accelerate the positive trajectory toward reducing the global epidemic to low endemic levels. This will require a strategic change of the AIDS response toward a long-term approach with some fundamental restructuring of current efforts.[20] Over the past three decades the AIDS movement has been able to overcome what seemed to be insurmountable obstacles. It still has the energy and creativity to take on this new challenge in the fight against what remains one of the greatest public health tragedies of modern times.

NOTES

INTRODUCTION

1. Marc Bloch, *The Historian's Craft,* trans. Peter Putnam (Manchester: Manchester University Press, 1992).
2. Peter Piot, *No Time to Lose: A Life in Pursuit of Deadly Viruses* (New York: W. W. Norton, 2012).
3. "Pneumocystis Pneumonia—Los Angeles," *CDC Morbidity and Mortality Weekly Report* 30 (1981): 250–252.
4. UNAIDS 2014, "Gap Report," http://www.unaids.org/en/resources/campaigns /2014/2014gapreport/gapreport/.
5. "Financing the Response to HIV in Low- and Middle-Income Countries: International Assistance from Donor Governments in 2013" (UNAIDS & The Henry J. Kaiser Family Foundation, 2014).
6. *AIDS at Thirty: Nations at the Crossroads* (Geneva: UNAIDS, 2011).
7. The aids2013 Consortium, *AIDS: Taking a Long-term View* (Upper Saddle River, NJ: Financial Times Science Press, 2010).
8. A. Jones et al., "Transformation of HIV from Pandemic to Low-Endemic Levels: A Public Health Approach to Combination Prevention," Lancet 384 (2014): 272–279.

1. A HETEROGENEOUS AND STILL-EVOLVING EPIDEMIC

1. P. Piot and T. C. Quinn, "Response to the AIDS Pandemic—A Global Health Model," *New England Journal of Medicine* 368 (2013): 2210–2218.
2. UNAIDS 2014, "Gap Report," http://www.unaids.org/en/resources/campaigns /2014/2014gapreport/gapreport/.
3. K. F. Ortblad, R. Lozano, and C. J. L. Murray, "The Burden of HIV: Insights from the Global Burden of Disease Study 2010," *AIDS* 27 (2013): 2003–2017.

4. "HIV Prevalence Estimates—United States, 2006," *CDC Morbidity and Mortality Weekly Report* 57 (2008): 1073–1076.

5. UNAIDS, *World AIDS Day Report* (Geneva: UNAIDS, 2012).

6. J. Chin, P. A. Sato, and J. M. Mann, "Projections of HIV Infections and AIDS Cases to the Year 2000," *Bulletin of the World Health Organization* 68 (1990): 1–11.

7. E. Gouws, V. Mishra, and T. B. Fowler, "Comparison of Adult HIV Prevalence from National Population-Based Surveys and Antenatal Clinic Surveillance in Countries with Generalised Epidemics: Implications for Calibrating Surveillance Data," *Sexually Transmitted Infections* 84 (2008): i17–i23.

8. H. G. Küstner, J. P. Swanevelder, and A. Van Middelkoop, "National HIV Surveillance—South Africa, 1990–1992," *South African Medical Journal* 84 (1994): 195–200.

9. See www.cdc.gov/nchhstp/stateprofiles/usmap.htm.

10. R. M. May and R. M. Anderson, "Transmission Dynamics of HIV Infection," *Nature* 326 (1987): 137–142.

11. K. Wellings et al., "Sexual Behaviour in Context: A Global Perspective," *Lancet* 368 (2006): 1706–1728.

12. T. B. Hallett et al., "Declines in HIV Prevalence Can Be Associated with Changing Sexual Behaviour in Uganda, Urban Kenya, Zimbabwe, and Urban Haiti," *Sexually Transmitted Infections* 82 (2006): i1–i8.

13. J. R. Glynn et al., "Why Do Young Women Have a Much Higher Prevalence of HIV than Young Men? A Study in Kisumu, Kenya and Ndola, Zambia," *AIDS* 15 (2001): S51–S60; K. M. Devries et al., "The Global Prevalence of Intimate Partner Violence Against Women," *Science* 340 (2013): 1527–1528.

2. HYPERENDEMIC HIV IN SOUTHERN AFRICA: THE HERITAGE OF APARTHEID

1. UNAIDS, *UNAIDS Report on the Global AIDS Epidemic* (Geneva: UNAIDS, 2013).

2. S. Gregson et al., "HIV Decline in Zimbabwe due to Reductions in Risky Sex? Evidence from a Comprehensive Epidemiological Review," *International Journal of Epidemiology* 39 (2010): 1311–1323.

3. R. Jewkes et al., "Factors Associated with HIV Sero-Status in Young Rural South African Women: Connections between Intimate Partner Violence and HIV," *International Journal of Epidemiology* 35 (2006): 1461–1468.

4. Q. Abdool Karim et al., "Effectiveness and Safety of Tenofovir Gel, an Antiretroviral Microbicide, for the Prevention of HIV Infection in Women," *Science* 329 (2010): 1168–1174.

5. B. Auvert et al., "Randomized, Controlled Intervention Trial of Male Circumcision for Reduction of HIV Infection Risk: The ANRS 1265 Trial," *PLoS Medicine* 2 (2005): e298.

6. M. Morris and M. Kretzschmar, "Concurrent Partnerships and the Spread of HIV," *AIDS* 11 (1997): 641–648.

7. G. Reniers and S. Watkins, "Polygyny and the Spread of HIV in Sub-Saharan Africa: A Case of Benign Concurrency," *AIDS* 24 (2010): 299–307.

8. Lesley Doyal and Imogen Pennell, *The Political Economy of Health* (London: Pluto Press, 1979).

9. Tamara Shefer et al., eds., *From Boys to Men: Social Constructions of Masculinity in Contemporary Society* (Landsdowne: University of Cape Town Press, 2007).

10. State of World Population 2005, "The Promise of Equality: Gender Equity, Reproductive Health and the Millennium Development Goals," United Nations Population Fund (UNFPA),

11. P. Piot, S. Russell, and H. Larson, "Good Politics, Bad Politics: The Experience of AIDS," *American Journal of Public Health* 97 (2007): 1934–1936.

12. Rob Dorrington et al., "The Impact of HIV/AIDS on Adult Mortality in South Africa," Technical Report (South African Medical Research Council, 2001).

13. N. Nattrass, "AIDS and the Scientific Governance of Medicine in Post-Apartheid South Africa," *African Affairs* 107 (2008): 157–176.

14. Hein Marais, *South Africa Pushed to the Limit: The Political Economy of Change* (London: Zed Books, 2011).

3. AIDS AS AN INTERNATIONAL POLITICAL ISSUE

1. Peter Piot, *No Time to Lose: A Life in Pursuit of Deadly Viruses* (New York: W. W. Norton, 2012).

2. Inge Kaul, I. Grunberg, and M. A. Stern, eds., *Global Public Goods: International Cooperation in the 21st Century* (New York: Oxford University Press, 1999). See also Inge Kaul et al., *Providing Global Public Goods: Managing Globalization* (New York: Oxford University Press, 2003).

3. UNAIDS 2009, "Denying Entry, Stay and Residence due to HIV Status," www.unaids. org/en/resources/documents/2009/name,33938,en.asp.

4. J. M. Mann, "Society and Public Health: Crisis and Rebirth," *Western Journal of Medicine* 169 (1998): 118–121.

5. S. Gruskin, E. J. Mills, and D. Tarantola, "History, Principles, and Practice of Health and Human Rights," *Lancet* 370 (2007): 449–455.

6. Mahbub ul Haq, *Reflections on Human Development* (New York: Oxford University Press, 1996), //hdr.undp.org/en/humandev/origins/.

7. See Mahbub ul Haq, http://hdr.undp.org/en/humandev/.

8. Barry Buzan, *People, States and Fear: An Agenda for International Security Studies in the Post-Cold War Era* (London: Harvester Wheatsheaf, 1991).

9. United Nations Security Council, 2000, "Resolution 1308," http://daccess-dds-ny. un.org/doc/UNDOC/GEN/N00/536/02/PDF/N0053602.pdf?OpenElement.

10. United Nations Economic and Social Council, 1995, "Paper E/1995/71," www.un.org /documents/ecosoc/docs/1995/e1995-71.htm.

11. United Nations Economic and Social Council, 1994, "Resolution 1994/24," www.unaids .org/en/media/unaids/contentassets/dataimport/pub/externaldocument/1994 /ecosoc_resolutions_establishing_unaids_en.pdf.

12. Lindsay Knight, *UNAIDS: The First 10 Years, 1996–2006* (Geneva: UNAIDS, 2008).

13. Noerine Kaleeba, *We Miss You All: AIDS in the Family* (Harare: Women and AIDS Support Network, 1991).

14. Malcolm Gladwell, *The Tipping Point: How Little Things Can Make a Big Difference* (Boston: Little, Brown 2000).

15. The Global Fund, 2013, www.theglobalfund.org/en/about/fundingspending/.

16. UNAIDS, *Drug Access Initiative* (Geneva: UNAIDS, 1998).

17. PEPFAR, "Funding and Results," http://www.pepfar.gov/funding/index.htm.

18. J. Shiffman and S. Smith, "Generation of Political Priority for Global Health Initiatives: A Framework and Case Study of Maternal Mortality," *Lancet* 370 (2007): 1370–1379.

4. A NEW TYPE OF TRANSNATIONAL CIVIL SOCIETY MOVEMENT

1. Social Watch Report 2010, *Time for a New Deal after the Fall* (Montevideo: Social Watch, 2010).

2. Michael Polanyi, *The Tacit Dimension* (London: Routledge and Kegan Paul, 1966).

3. R. G. Parker, "Civil Society, Political Mobilization, and the Impact of HIV Scale-Up on Health Systems in Brazil," *Journal of Acquired Immune Deficiency Syndromes* 52 (2009): suppl. 1, S49–51.

4. M. Heywood, "South Africa's Treatment Action Campaign: Combining Law and Social Mobilization to Realize the Right to Health," *Journal of Human Rights Practice* 1 (2009): 14–36.

5. S. Tantivess and G. Walt, "The Role of State and Non-State Actors in the Policy Process: The Contribution of Policy Networks to the Scale-Up of Antiretroviral Therapy in Thailand," *Health Policy and Planning* 23 (2008): 328–338.

6. A. Appadurai, "Grassroots Globalization and the Research Imagination," *Public Culture* 12 (2000): 1–19.

7. Françoise Héritier, "Les Matrices de l'Intolérance et de la Violence," in *De la Violence II: Séminaire de Françoise Héritier* ed. F. Héritier (Paris: Odile Jacob, 1999).

8. E. H. McWhirter, "Empowerment in Counseling," *Journal of Counseling and Development* 69 (1991): 222–227.

5. THE RIGHT TO TREATMENT

1. J. G. Bartlett, "Ten Years of HAART: Foundation for the Future," *Medscape* (2006), www.medscape.org/viewarticle/523119.

2. D. Trono et al., "HIV Persistence and the Prospect of Long-Term Drug-Free Remissions for HIV-Infected Individuals," *Science* 329 (2010): 174–180.

3. P. Mugyenyi et al., "Scaling Up Antiretroviral Therapy: Experience of the Joint Clinical Research Centre (JCRC) Access Programme," *Acta Academica* (2006), suppl. 1: 216–240 (http://reference.sabinet.co.za/sa_epublication_article/academ _supp1_2006_a9).

4. "Each Member has the right to determine what constitutes a national emergency or other circumstances of extreme urgency, it being understood that public health crises, including those relating to HIV/AIDS, tuberculosis, malaria and other epidemics, can represent a national emergency or other circumstances of extreme urgency." Doha Declaration, paragraph 5.

5. B. Schwartländer et al., "AIDS: Resource needs for HIV/AIDS," *Science* 292 (2001): 2434–2436.

6. UNAIDS 2014, "Gap Report," http://www.unaids.org/en/resources/campaigns /2014/2014gapreport/gapreport/.

7. Panel on Antiretroviral Guidelines for Adults and Adolescents, *Guidelines for the Use of Antiretroviral Agents in HIV-1-Infected Adults and Adolescents* (Washington DC: Department of Health and Human Services, 2012 [updated 2013]); *Consolidated Guidelines on the Use of Antiretroviral Drugs for Treating and Preventing HIV Infection* (Geneva: World Health Organization, 2013); D. D. Ho, "Time to Hit HIV, Early and Hard," *New England Journal of Medicine* 333 (1995): 450–451; T. W. Chun and A. S. Fauci "Latent Reservoirs of HIV: Obstacles to the Eradication of Virus," *Proceedings of the National Academy of Sciences* 96 (1999): 10958–10961.

8. *Guidelines Version 6.1* (Paris: European AIDS Clinical Society, 2012); Williams, I et al., "British HIV Association Guidelines for the Treatment of HIV-1-Positive Adults with Antiretroviral Therapy 2012," *HIV Medicine* 15 (2014): 1–6.

9. M. S. Cohen et al., "Prevention of HIV-1 Infection with Early Antiretroviral Therapy," *New England Journal of Medicine* 365 (2011): 493–505.

10. A. Gupta et al., "Early Mortality in Adults Initiating Antiretroviral Therapy (ART) in Low-and Middle-Income Countries (LMIC): A Systematic Review and Meta-Analysis," *PLoS One* 6 (2011): e28691.

11. A. Boulle et al., "Seven-Year Experience of a Primary Care Antiretroviral Treatment Programme in Khayelitsha, South Africa," *AIDS* 24 (2010): 563–572.

12. M. May et al., "Prognosis of HIV-1 Infected Patients Starting Antiretroviral Therapy in Sub-Saharan Africa: A Collaborative Analysis of Scale-Up Programmes," *Lancet* 376 (2010): 449–457.

13. UNAIDS, *Global Report: UNAIDS Report on the Global AIDS Epidemic 2012* (Geneva: UNAIDS, 2012).

14. M. Piot, *A Simulation Model of Case Finding and Treatment in Tuberculosis Control Programmes* (Geneva: World Health Organization, 1967).

15. J. Y. Kim, P. Farmer, and M. E. Porter, "Redefining Global Health-Care Delivery," *Lancet* 382 (2013): 1060–1069.

16. S. D. Foster et al., "The Experience of 'Medicine Companions' to Support Adherence to Antiretroviral Therapy: Quantitative and Qualitative Data from a Trial Population in Uganda," *AIDS Care* 22 (2010), suppl. 1: 35–43.

17. S. Jaffar et al., "Rates of Virological Failure in Patients Treated in a Home-Based Versus a Facility-Based HIV-Care Model in Jinja, Southeast Uganda: A Cluster-Randomised Equivalence Trial," *Lancet* 374 (2009): 2080–2089.

18. DART Trial Team, "Routine Versus Clinically Driven Laboratory Monitoring of HIV Antiretroviral Therapy in Africa (DART): A Randomised Non-Inferiority Trial," *Lancet* 375 (2010): 123–131.

19. E. B. Kapstein and J. W. Busby, *AIDS Drugs for All: Social Movements and Market Transformation* (Cambridge: Cambridge University Press, 2013).

6. COMBINATION PREVENTION

1. A. S. Fauci, "An AIDS-Free Generation Is Closer than We Might Think," *Washington Post* July 12, 2013.

2. Q. Abdool Karim et al., "Effectiveness and Safety of Tenofovir Gel, an Antiretroviral Microbicide, for the Prevention of HIV Infection in Women," *Science* 329 (2010): 1168–1174.

3. R. M. Grant et al., "Preexposure Chemoprophylaxis for HIV Prevention in Men Who Have Sex with Men," *New England Journal of Medicine* 363 (2010): 2587–2599.

4. R. M. May and R. M. Anderson, "Transmission Dynamics of HIV Infection," *Nature* 326 (1987): 137–142.

5. UNAIDS, *UNAIDS World AIDS Day Report* (Geneva: UNAIDS, 2012).

6. UNAIDS, *UNAIDS Report on the Global AIDS Epidemic* (Geneva: UNAIDS, 2010).

7. T. B. Hallett et al., "Declines in HIV Prevalence Can Be Associated with Changing Sexual Behaviour in Uganda, Urban Kenya, Zimbabwe, and Urban Haiti," *Sexually Transmitted Infections* 82 (2006): i1–i8; T. B. Hallett et al., "Assessing Evidence for Behaviour Change Affecting the Course of HIV Epidemics: A New Mathematical Modelling Approach and Application to Data from Zimbabwe," *Epidemics* 1 (2009): 108–117.

8. M. Potts et al., "Reassessing HIV Prevention," *Science* 320 (2008): 749–750.

9. Helen Epstein, *The Invisible Cure: Africa, the West, and the Fight against AIDS* (London: Penguin, 2007).

10. J. S. G. Montaner et al., "The Case for Expanding Access to Highly Active Antiretroviral Therapy to Curb the Growth of the HIV Epidemic," *Lancet* 368 (2006): 531–536 ; K. M. De Cock et al., "Can Antiretroviral Therapy Eliminate HIV Transmission?" *Lancet* 373 (2009): 7–9.

11. P. Piot et al., "Coming to Terms with Complexity: A Call to Action for HIV Prevention," *Lancet* 372 (2008): 845–859.

12. E. Duflo et al., "Education and HIV/AIDS Prevention: Evidence from a Randomized Evaluation in Western Kenya" (World Bank Policy Research Working Paper 4024, 2006).

13. UNESCO, SIDALAC, PAHO Report of AIDS Cases, 2010.

14. C. Beyrer et al., "The Expanding Epidemics of HIV Type 1 among Men Who Have Sex with Men in Low- and Middle-Income Countries: Diversity and Consistency," Epidemiologic Reviews 32 (2010): 137–151.

15. M. S. Cohen et al., "Prevention of HIV-1 Iinfection with Early Antiretroviral Therapy," New England Journal of Medicine 365 (2011): 493–505.

16. T. C. Quinn et al., "Viral Load and Heterosexual Transmission of Human Immunodeficiency Virus Type 1," New England Journal of Medicine 342 (2000): 921–929.

17. J. Birungi et al., "Lack of Effectiveness of Antiretroviral Therapy (ART) as an HIV Prevention Tool for Discordant Couples in Rural ART Program without Viral Load Monitoring in Uganda" (19th International AIDS Conference, Washington, DC, Abstract TUAC0103, 2013).

18. Q. Abdool Karim et al., "Effectiveness and Safety of Tenofovir Gel, an Antiretroviral Microbicide, for the Prevention of HIV Infection in Women," Science 329 (2010): 1168–1174.

19. P. Piot and T. C. Quinn, "Response to the AIDS Pandemic—A Global Health Model," New England Journal of Medicine 368 (2013): 2210–2218.

20. B. Auvert et al., "Randomized, Controlled Intervention Trial of Male Circumcision for Reduction of HIV Infection Risk: The ANRS 1265 Trial," PLoS Medicine 2 (2005): e298.

21. D. W. Cameron et al., "Female to Male Transmission of Human Immunodeficiency Virus Type 1: Risk Factors for Seroconversion in Men," Lancet 2 (1989): 403–407.

22. E. M. Connor et al., "Reduction of Maternal-Infant Transmission of Human Immunodeficiency Virus Type 1 with Zidovudine Treatment," New England Journal of Medicine 331 (1994): 1173–1180.

23. World Health Organization, Consolidated Guidelines on the Use of Antiretroviral Drugs for Treating and Preventing HIV Infection: Recommendations for a Public Health Approach (Geneva: World Health Organization, 2013).

24. UNAIDS 2014, "Gap Report," http://www.unaids.org/en/resources/campaigns/2014/2014gapreport/gapreport/.

25. Committee on the Prevention of HIV Infection among Injecting Drug Users in High-Risk Countries, Preventing HIV Infection among Injecting Drug Users in High-Risk Countries: An Assessment of the Evidence (Washington: The National Academies Press, 2006).

26. Human Rights Watch and the International Harm Reduction Association, Drugs, Punitive Laws, Policies, and Policing Practices, and HIV/AIDS, 2009 (http://www.hrw.org/fr/news/2009/11/30/drugs-punitive-laws-policies-and-policing-practices-and-hivaids).

27. P. Piot, S. Russell, and H. Larson, "Good Politics, Bad Politics: The Experience of AIDS," *American Journal of Public Health* 97 (2007): 1934–1936.

28. R. Doll and A. B. Hill, "Smoking and Carcinoma of the Lung," *British Medical Journal* 2 (1950): 739–748.

29. G. R. Gupta et al., "Structural Approaches to HIV Prevention," *Lancet* 372 (2008): 764–775.

30. K. M. Devries et al., "The Global Prevalence of Intimate Partner Violence against Women," *Science* 340 (2013): 1527–1528.

31. R. K. Jewkes et al., "Intimate Partner Violence, Relationship Power Inequity, and Incidence of HIV Infection in Young Women in South Africa: A Cohort Study," *Lancet* 376 (2010): 41–48.

32. S. Baird et al., "The Short-Term Impacts of a Schooling Conditional Cash Transfer Program on the Sexual Behavior of Young Women," *Health Economics* 19 (2010): suppl. 55–68.

33. P. M. Pronyk et al., "Effect of a Structural Intervention for the Prevention of Intimate-Partner Violence and HIV in Rural South Africa: A Cluster Randomised Trial," *Lancet* 368 (2006): 1973–1983.

34. E. Duflo et al., "Education and HIV/AIDS Prevention: Evidence from a Randomized Evaluation in Western Kenya" (World Bank Policy Research Working Paper 4024, 2006).

35. S. M. Bertozzi et al., "Making HIV Prevention Programmes Work," *Lancet* 372 (2008): 831–844.

36. Global Commission on HIV and the Law, *HIV and the Law: Risks, Rights & Health* (New York: UN Development Programme, 2012).

37. J. Esparza, "A Brief History of the Global Effort to Develop a Preventive HIV Vaccine," *Vaccine* 31 (2013): 3502–3518.

38. A. Jones et al., "Transformation of HIV from Pandemic to Low-Endemic Levels: A Public Health Approach to Combination Prevention," *Lancet* 384 (2014): 272–279.

7. THE ECONOMICS OF AIDS

1. P. Piot, R. Greener, and S. Russell, "Squaring the Circle: AIDS, Poverty, and Human Development," *PLoS Medicine* 4 (2007): e314.

2. M. Over, *The Macroeconomic Impact of AIDS in Sub-Saharan Africa* (Washington, DC: World Bank Population Health and Nutrition Division, 1992).

3. International Labour Organization, *HIV/AIDS and Work: Global Estimates, Impact and Response* (Geneva: International Labour Office, 2004).

4. M. Over et al., *Coping with AIDS: The Economic Impact of Adult Mortality from AIDS and Other Causes on Households in Kagera, Tanzania* (Washington, DC: World Bank, 1996).

5. A. Ilinigumugabo, "The Economic Consequences of AIDS in Africa," *African Journal of Fertility, Sexuality and Reproductive Health* 1 (1996): 153–161.

6. D. T. Jamison et al., "Global Health 2035: A World Converging within a Generation," *Lancet* 382 (2013): 1898–1955

7. B. Schwartländer et al., "Towards an Improved Investment Approach for an Effective Response to HIV/AIDS," *Lancet* 377 (2011): 2031–2041.

8. R. Hecht et al., "Critical Choices in Financing the Response to the Global HIV/AIDS Pandemic," *Health Affairs* 28 (2009): 1591–1605.

9. Transparency International, *Global Corruption Report 2006* (London: Pluto Press, 2006).

10. R. Lozano et al., "Global and Regional Mortality from 235 Causes of Death for 20 Age Groups in 1990 and 2010: A Systematic Analysis for the Global Burden of Disease Study 2010," *Lancet* 380 (2013): 2095–2128. Additional data from www.healthmetricsandevaluation.org/gbd.

11. A. Jones et al., "Transformation of HIV from Pandemic to Low-Endemic Levels: A Public Health Approach to Combination Prevention," *Lancet* 384 (2014): 272–279.

12. Disability Adjusted Life Years (DALYs) is an indicator used for quantifying the burden of disease from mortality and morbidity. One DALY can be thought of as one lost year of "healthy" life.

13. O. Galárraga et al., "HIV Prevention Cost-Effectiveness: A Systematic Review," *BMC Public Health* 9 (2009), suppl. 1: S5.

14. M. Over et al., "Antiretroviral Therapy and HIV Prevention in India: Modeling Costs and Consequences of Policy Options," *Sexually Transmitted Diseases* 33 (2006): S145–S152.

15. M. Khobotlo et al., http://siteresources.worldbank.org/INTHIVAIDS/Resources /375798-1103037153392/LesothoMOT13April.pdf (2009).

16. R. Hecht et al., "Critical Choices in Financing the Response to the Global HIV/AIDS Pandemic," *Health Affairs* 28 (2009): 1591–1605.

17. A. Vassall et al., "Financing Essential HIV Services: A New Economic Agenda," *PLoS Medicine* 10 (2013): e1001567.

8. PROMINENCE OF HUMAN RIGHTS

1. J. M. Mann, Statement at an Informal Briefing on AIDS to the 42nd Session of the United Nations General Assembly, October 20, 1987, New York.

2. Katarina Tomasevski et al., "AIDS and Human Rights," in *AIDS in the World*, vol. 1, ed. J. Mann, D. J. M. Tarantola, T. W. Netter (Cambridge: Harvard University Press, 1992).

3. J. Mann and D. J. M. Tarantola, eds., *AIDS in the World*, vol. 2 (New York: Oxford University Press, 1996).

4. *Protocol for the Identification of Discrimination against People Living with HIV* (Geneva: UNAIDS, 2000).

5. Susan Sontag, *AIDS and Its Metaphors* (New York: Farrar, Straus and Giroux, 1989).

6. Michel Foucault, *History of Madness*, trans. J. Khalfa and J. Murphy (London: Routledge, 2006).

7. Mirko D. Grmek, *History of AIDS: Emergence and Origin of a Modern Pandemic* (Princeton: Princeton University Press, 1993).

8. Michel Foucault, *The History of Sexuality*, vol. 2: *The Use of Pleasure*, trans. Robert Hurley (New York: Pantheon, 1985).

9. Germaine Brée, *Camus* (New Brunswick: Rutgers University Press, 1961).

10. ICRW, *Understanding HIV-Related Stigma and Resulting Discrimination in Sub-Saharan Africa* (Washington, DC: International Center for Research on Women, 2002).

11. Erving Goffman, *Stigma: Notes on the Management of Spoiled Identity* (New York: Simon and Schuster, 1963).

12. K. M. Devries et al., "The Global Prevalence of Intimate Partner Violence against Women," *Science* 340 (2013): 1527–1528.

13. J. C. Campbell et al., "The Intersection of Intimate Partner Violence against Women and HIV/AIDS: A Review," *International Journal of Injury Control and Safety Promotion* 15 (2008): 221–231; R. K. Jewkes et al., "Intimate Partner Violence, Relationship Power Inequity, and Incidence of HIV Infection in Young Women in South Africa: A Cohort Study," *Lancet* 376 (2010): 41–48.

14. S. L. Martin et al., "Sexual Behaviors and Reproductive Health Outcomes: Associations with Wife Abuse in India," *Journal of the American Medical Association* 282 (1999): 1967–1972.

15. Daniel Ottosson, *State-Sponsored Homophobia* (Brussels: International Lesbian, Gay, Bisexual, Trans and Intersex Association, 2010).

16. *The China Stigma Index Report* (Geneva: UNAIDS, 2009).

17. L. Stackpool-Moore et al., "Give Stigma the Index Finger! Results from *The People Living with HIV Stigma Index* in the UK in 2009" (THPE0938, Vienna: International AIDS Conference, 2010).

18. S. Paxton et al., "AIDS-related Discrimination in Asia," *AIDS Care* 17 (2005): 413–424.

19. "Each Member has the right to determine what constitutes a national emergency or other circumstances of extreme urgency, it being understood that public health crises, including those relating to HIV/AIDS, tuberculosis, malaria and other epidemics, can represent a national emergency or other circumstances of extreme urgency." Doha declaration, article 5.

20. Jürgen Habermas, *The Structural Transformation of the Public Sphere: An Inquiry into a Category of Bourgeois Society* (Cambridge: Polity, 1989).

21. Global Commission on HIV and the Law, *HIV and the Law: Risks, Rights & Health*, (New York: UN Development Programme, 2012).

22. Office of the United Nations High Commissioner for Human Rights, *International Guidelines on HIV/AIDS and Human Rights* (Geneva: UNAIDS, 2006).

23. E. Cameron, "HIV is a Virus, Not a Crime: Criminal Statutes and Criminal Prosecutions" (FRPL0103, Mexico: International AIDS Conference, 2008).

9. THE LONG-TERM VIEW

1. Oxford Martin Commission for Future Generations, *Now for the Long Term* (Oxford: Oxford Martin School, 2013).

2. R. M. Granich et al., "Universal Voluntary HIV Testing with Immediate Antiretroviral Therapy as a Strategy for Elimination of HIV Transmission: A Mathematical Model," *Lancet* 373 (2009): 48–57.

3. C. Beyrer et al., "Time to Act: A Call for Comprehensive Responses to HIV in People Who Use Drugs," *Lancet* 376 (2010): 551–563; C. Beyrer et al., Global Epidemiology of HIV Infection among Men Who Have Sex with Men," *Lancet* 380 (2012): 367–377; S. Baral et al., "Burden of HIV among Female Sex Workers in Low-Income and Middle-Income Countries: A Systematic Review and Meta-Analysis," *Lancet Infectious Diseases* 12 (2012): 538–549.

4. The aids2031 Consortium, *AIDS: Taking a Long-term View* (Upper Saddle River, NJ: Financial Times Science Press, 2010).

5. L. S. Zabin et al., "Levels of Change in Adolescent Sexual Behavior in Three Asian Cities," *Studies in Family Planning* 40 (2009): 1–12.

6. C. H. Mercer et al., "Changes in Sexual Attitudes and Lifestyles in Britain through the Life Course and Over Time: Findings from the National Surveys of Sexual Attitudes and Lifestyles (Natsal)," *Lancet* 382 (2013): 1781–1794.

7. S. M. Bertozzi, T. E. Martz, and P. Piot, "The Evolving HIV/AIDS Response and the Urgent Tasks Ahead," *Health Affairs* 28 (2009): 1578–1590; The aids2031 Consortium, *AIDS: Taking a Long-term View* (Upper Saddle River, NJ: Financial Times Science Press, 2010).

8. A. Jones et al., "Transformation of HIV from Pandemic to Low-Endemic Levels: A Public Health Approach to Combination Prevention," *Lancet* 384 (2014): 272–279.

9. M. A. Boyd and D. A. Cooper, "Optimisation of HIV Care and Service Delivery: Doing More with Less," *Lancet* 380 (2012): 1860–1866.

10. R. Hecht et al., "Critical Choices in Financing the Response to the Global HIV/AIDS Pandemic," *Health Affairs* 28 (2009): 1591–1605.

11. E. Lule and M. Haacker, *The Fiscal Dimension of HIV/AIDS in Botswana, South Africa, Swaziland, and Uganda* (Washington, DC: The World Bank, 2011).

12. B. Schwartländer et al., "Towards an Improved Investment Approach for an Effective Response to HIV/AIDS," *Lancet* 377 (2011): 2031–2041.

13. D. T. Jamison et al., "Global Health 2035: A World Converging within a Generation," *Lancet* 382 (2013): 1898–1955.

14. A. Vassall et al., "Financing Essential HIV Services: A New Economic Agenda," *PLoS Medicine* 10, no. 12 (2013): e1001567.

15. S. M. Bertozzi, T. E. Martz, and P. Piot, "The Evolving HIV/AIDS Response and the Urgent Tasks Ahead," *Health Affairs* 28 (2009): 1578–1590.

16. J. Y. Kim, P. Farmer, and M. E. Porter, "Redefining Global Health-Care Delivery," *Lancet* 382 (2013): 1060–1069.

17. J. Esparza, "A Brief History of the Global Effort to Develop a Preventive HIV Vaccine," *Vaccine* 31 (2013): 3502–3518.

18. S. Rerks-Ngarm et al., "Vaccination with ALVAC and AIDSVAX to Prevent HIV-1 Infection in Thailand," *New England Journal of Medicine* 361 (2009): 2209–2220.

19. A. S. Fauci, "An AIDS-Free Generation Is Closer than We Might Think," *Washington Post*, July 12, 2013.

20. H. J. Larson, S. Bertozzi, and P. Piot, "Redesigning the AIDS Response for Long-Term Impact," *Bulletin of the World Health Organization* 89 (2011): 846–821.

INDEX

Abuja Declaration, 141

Accelerating Access Initiative, UNAIDS-WHO, 96–97

Access Campaign, MSF, 93

accountability, transnational civil society movements, 85

Achmat, Zackie, 43–44, 80, 81

activism, AIDS-related, 3; AIDS and globalization, 82–88; conditions for success of, 72–73; fundamental role of in AIDS response, 76–82; heterogeneity of activism, 77–82; in long-term approach to AIDS, 168–169; overview, 74–76; transnational civil society movements, 84–86

ACT UP, 78

ACT UP France, 77

addiction treatment, 123–125

adherence, treatment, 104–105

advocacy, by transnational civil society movements, 85. *See also* activism, AIDS-related

Africa: AIDS-related deaths in, 17; AIDS response in, 60–61; declines in HIV incidence in, 111–112; demonstrating feasibility of antiretrovirals in, 92–94; diversification of epidemics in, 14–15, 22; economic drivers of AIDS, 131–133; male

circumcision in, 121; mother-to-child transmission, preventing, 123; need for international financing in, 139; orphans in, 136–137; overlap between high-risk groups and geography, 116–117; penal laws specific to HIV in, 159; prevention efforts for high-risk populations, 117; productivity and services, impact of AIDS on, 137–138; regional AIDS initiatives in, 67–68; transmission patterns in, 113; treatment adherence in, 105; treatment challenges, 106; treatment coverage in, 101. *See also* hyperendemic HIV in Southern Africa; *specific countries*

ageing processes, accelerated, 105

AIDES organization, 77

aids2031 Consortium, 128, 161–162

AIDS and Its Metaphors, 149

"AIDS in the workplace" programs, 65

AIDS Law Project, 80–81

AIDS movement, 3; AIDS and globalization, 82–88; conditions for success of, 72–73; fundamental role of in AIDS response, 76–82; heterogeneity of activism, 77–82; long-term approach to AIDS, 168–169; overview, 74–76; transnational civil society movements, 84–86